Praise for *Rest, Play, Grow*

"This book is a tribute to not only Dr. MacNamara's giftedness but also to her absolute driving conviction that the insights regarding relationship and development must get out to those who are responsible for raising our youngsters… Dr. MacNamara is wonderfully positioned to tell you this story, taking you from theory to practice. You could not be in better hands."

—GORDON NEUFELD, PhD, bestselling author and founder of the Neufeld Institute

"Deborah MacNamara's book is rich with insights into both the nature of the child and positive parenting. A boon to parents and teachers, *Rest, Play, Grow* notes the preeminence of early parent-child attachment in optimal development, and it passionately affirms the primary value of play to children's well-being and creativity. Dr. MacNamara is highly attuned to both children's needs and parental best practices. Read, reflect, share."

—RAFFI CAVOUKIAN, CM, singer, author, and founder of the Centre for Child Honouring

"Basing her approach in attachment theory and the groundbreaking work of Dr. Gordon Neufeld, Deborah MacNamara has written an essential primer on how to be a parent by making sense of the inner world of children. This book is developmental science translated into practical love."

—GABOR MATÉ, MD, co-author of *Hold On to Your Kids*

"This is a must-read for every parent of a preschooler or younger. Dr. MacNamara clearly shows the developmental stages of preschoolers so that parents gain a better understanding of the emotional state of the child. It is with this understanding that parenting the preschooler becomes easier. Read this and you will truly be your 'kid's best bet.'"

—KRISTY PILLINGER, editor-in-chief of *Nurture Parenting Magazine*

"Reading *Rest, Play, Grow* brought me to tears because it reaffirmed my gut instincts as a parent. Dr. MacNamara translates a child's language and maturity into an understandable framework, which will you give you that 'aha' moment while reading it, and then she supports you with practices to manage the big emotions of children. *Rest, Play, Grow* combines real science with real-life stories, humour, and sensible strategies. Deborah has translated the beautifully chaotic world of being a preschooler. If there is only one book you should read as a parent, this is the one."

—TRACI COSTA, CEO of Peek…

"As a practicing pediatrician, I spend much of my day listening to parental concerns about their toddlers' imperfections. 'How can I get my child to eat more, sleep better, toilet train faster, behave reasonably, and be smart but not outsmart me?' I think of my dear friend Dr. MacNamara and ask myself, 'How would she answer this question?' I am delighted that she has put those answers in this wonderful book, full of developmental wisdom and practical advice on the daily life of maturing toddlers and their evolving parents. This is not a quick-fix script but, instead, presents a road map to better understand this amazing age in all its glorious imperfections."

—**KEYVAN HADAD,** MD, medical director, Intermediate Nursery, BC Women's Hospital; clinical associate professor, University of British Columbia

"*Rest, Play, Grow* is a refreshing reminder of the importance of slowing down and allowing children to mature at their own pace, unhindered by societal expectations. With insight and sensitivity, Dr. MacNamara guides parents to trust their intuition to provide the conditions for children to grow rather than offering tools for changing behavior. After reading Dr. Deborah MacNamara's book, embracing a child's immaturity has never felt so fulfilling or freeing."

—**LORI PETRO,** founder of TEACH through Love

"Dr. MacNamara's beautifully written book gently expands the reader's perspective, providing a different lens for viewing the child, one that both widens and deepens understanding. Bringing richness to Dr. Neufeld's words and models, she helps the reader to do the work of applying such important theory with their own family. Dr. MacNamara truly has the gift of writing, always grounding concepts in very relatable moments from her life and work as a researcher, professor, counsellor, and, of course, parent."

—**GENEVIEVE SIMPERINGHAM,** co-founder of the Peaceful Parent Institute

"Finally, a book for parents of young children that weds neuroscience and attachment research and is consummately useful! I am certain that *Rest, Play, Grow* will be the go-to guide for confused and exhausted parents who are receiving mixed messages from professionals and the culture-at-large about how to raise their children. Dr. MacNamara shows us what we have sensed all along: the answers are within us, and we parents are the relationship experts we have been looking for. I guarantee you that *Rest, Play, Grow* will be your parenting training wheels, and that by book's end you will be navigating your parenting journey with the utmost skill, confidence, and joy!"

—**SIL REYNOLDS,** co-author of *Mothering & Daughtering: Keeping Your Bond Strong through the Teen Years*

Rest, Play, Grow

foreword by **GORDON NEUFELD, PhD**

DEBORAH MACNAMARA, PhD

REST
PLAY
GROW

Making Sense of Preschoolers
(Or Anyone Who Acts Like One)

Based on the relational developmental approach of Gordon Neufeld

For Chris, Hannah, and Madeline,
because we rest, play, and grow together.

. . . .

19 20 21 22 7 6 5 4

Aona Books
Vancouver, Canada

Cataloguing data available from Library and Archives Canada
ISBN 978-0-9950512-0-1 (paperback)
ISBN 978-0-9950512-1-8 (ebook)

http://macnamara.ca/

Based on the relational developmental approach of Gordon Neufeld

Editing by Shirarose Wilensky
Copyediting by Stephanie Fysh
Proofreading by Lana Okerlund
Cover and interior design by Nayeli Jimenez
Cover photograph by iStockphoto.com
Interior images courtesy of Dr. Gordon Neufeld

Names have been changed unless specific permission to use them has
been granted by the individual.

Printed in Canada

"Please do not torment, pester, worry, badger, harry, harass, heckle, persecute, irk, bully, vex, disquiet, grate, beset, tease, nettle, or tantalize the young children."

(Adapted from the San Diego Zoo guidelines
for the treatment of animals)

Contents

Foreword

AN ENCOUNTER WITH Dr. MacNamara is not soon to be forgotten.
She is a dynamo of energy, intellect, and wit, seizing most any situation by storm, albeit the calmest kind of storm you can imagine. She
certainly has a profound effect, though she often looks the picture of
serenity. I have always found that to be a rather remarkable achievement—one I'm sure her children must benefit from immensely.

Our relationship began as student and teacher. Deborah was
quick to grasp developmental theory, as well as to realize the implications of an attachment-based approach to parenting. As soon as
she understood the power of these insights, she insisted that they
needed to be shared widely, and I am delighted that she has chosen
to take up this role.

Deborah's mastery of attachment and development theory has
been impressive. But what impressed me most in the early days of
our relationship was her groundedness with the material. She seemed
to have an intuitive sense of the transition from theory to practice.
While holding on to the big picture, she was able to bring the material to the most concrete of applications. While I was still in my head,
she had moved to a myriad of practical applications. Yet she didn't
get lost in the details or go down the many potential rabbit holes.

Our roles have reversed somewhat from those early days. More
often than not, she is the one now taking the lead, scouring the

scientific literature for relevant material and breaking research, and turning my head when she comes across material that she thinks I should read. Deborah knows what is current in developmental science and understands her ultimate accountability to the scientific pursuit of truth. A critical mind and a scientific bent are essential tools when attempting to make sense of things, especially complex phenomena such as attachment and immaturity.

I also appreciate the theorist in Deborah. I have laid some of the foundations of the attachment-based developmental approach, but she has shown her creative brilliance in building on this material, taking it a step further, opening some doors before me.

Parenting the preschooler is not an easy task. How do you keep the attachment in mind, create a sense of security, retain your caring alpha lead, provide a sense of rest, yet know when to draw the line and invite the tears—all in the very same dance? Many devoted parents, even when equipped with insight, err too much in one direction or the other. Some parents become rather indulgent and lose their lead, giving rise to anxious alpha-type children who need to be in control. These parents do nurturance well but cannot provide the containment and the walls of futility that are absolutely needed for healthy development to occur. Other parents can take the lead all right, assuming their role as agents of adaptation, but have difficulty getting their love across when they are feeling frustrated.

Deborah found a way through, and that, to my mind, is her most significant qualification for writing about young children. Theoretical mastery is not enough when it comes to teaching others. One needs to have incorporated this knowledge into the kind of dance that allows nature to have its wonderful way with our children.

Two themes pervade this book. The first is the importance of the relationship—the right kind of relationship—for bringing children to their full potential as human beings. We must never forget that it is the child's relationship to the parent or teacher that is the natural context for raising that child. When there are problems in the relationship, such as resistance to proximity or the child being in the lead, nothing will work quite right. In the past, culture protected relationships through rituals and customs. This, sadly, is no longer the case, hence the need for consciousness of the relational factor. It turns out that the preschooler period is absolutely pivotal in developing the capacity for relationship. Nothing could be more important than this factor in development. We must always keep attachment in mind.

The second theme is immaturity. One would think that the fact that preschoolers are immature would be self-evident. On the contrary, immaturity is one of the most neglected and misunderstood constructs today. What Piaget discovered—that immaturity renders the preschooler a fundamentally different creature—has never quite hit our consciousness, at least not enough to make a difference in our dance. If we truly understood immaturity, we would not be tripping all over our preschoolers. If we truly understood immaturity, we would not think it a flaw that requires correction. If we truly understood immaturity, we would not punish a child for being immature. It turns out that there is a very good reason for immaturity: it is part of the developmental design.

The fundamental human problem is that we don't all grow up as we grow older. This stuckness often begins as a youngster. Preschoolers certainly have a right to their immaturity; the problem arises when we are still acting like preschoolers when we are no longer that age. The more we understand about the immaturity of a preschooler—what is missing and why—the more we can appreciate the conditions that are conducive to true maturation, the less we will trip over our preschoolers, and the more we can take up a relationship with our own immaturity. Immaturity is immaturity, no matter how old we are.

It may seem rather ironic, but I believe that today's parents are for the most part taking far too much responsibility for raising their children. We are forgetting that maturation happened long before there were any books, long before there were any teachers, long before we had any inkling of how maturation happened, long before there were schools, long before there was therapy. The good news is that if a parent really gets the message of this book, there will be an appreciation of the developmental process that can put them at ease. We don't have to push the river, as most of us have become preoccupied with doing. If we know what nature requires to do its job and can provide those conditions, we can afford to relax somewhat and then celebrate the spontaneous fruit that will result.

I was so pleased when Deborah announced to me—a few years ago now—her intentions to write a book on making sense of the preschooler. Her two young girls had provided her with a treasure trove of illustrations and anecdotes. But how to find the space and the time to do this? Her giftedness as a presenter had made her much in demand as a speaker at conferences and professional development workshops. Her devotion as a parent meant that she was not prepared to compromise herself in this arena. This book is a tribute not only to her giftedness but also to her absolute driving conviction that the insights regarding relationship and development must get out to those who are responsible for raising our youngsters. In an attempt to create some space for this, she had already quit her day job teaching at university. She had also cut back her private practice. Without this unstoppable drive and the corresponding sacrifices she was willing to make, this book would never have materialized. Deborah is wonderfully positioned to tell this story, taking you from theory to practice. You could not be in better hands.

DR. GORDON NEUFELD

Introduction
Why Making Sense Matters

---

*To understand a child we have to watch him at play, study
him in his different moods; we cannot project upon him our own
prejudices, hopes and fears, or mould him to fit the pattern
of our desires. If we are constantly judging the child according to our
personal likes and dislikes, we are bound to create barriers
and hindrances in our relationship with him and in his
relationships with the world.*
JIDDU KRISHNAMURTI[1]

A NUMBER OF YEARS ago, I was invited to speak to a group of
new parents on the subject of attachment and young children.
The room at the community centre was crammed with mothers nursing their babies, rocking them to sleep, or changing their
diapers. Car carriers, strollers, and baby bags were piled on top of
each other, all with blankets bursting forth. Meredith, the coordinator of the weekly support group, invited the parents to sit on chairs
arranged in a circle. She began her check-in with a warm welcome
and asked everyone how they were managing. A number of parents
replied that they were getting out of the house, some said they had
managed to take a shower, and others replied that breastfeeding was
going better. A tired-looking mother spoke up and said, "My baby
cries every time I put her down. I nurse her until she falls asleep,

but as soon as I put her in the crib, she wakes up. I'm so exhausted." There were nods and sighs of agreement as Meredith responded, "Yes, it is hard. You just want some rest and they always seem to need you." More nods of agreement ensued as Meredith paused before continuing, "I imagine it is hard for your baby, too. They are transitioning from being inside you 24/7, feeling your warmth, hearing your heartbeat, to never being able to hold you close like that again." The room was silent for a moment and I found myself travelling back to when I first became a parent. I began to feel the mothers' apprehension, excitement, and exhaustion viscerally.

Meredith then formally welcomed me to the parent group and introduced me as someone she had invited to speak on the topic of attachment. She emphasized to the mothers the importance of human relationships and said this process of attachment was already unfolding between them and their babies. She had forewarned me that I would have 15 minutes to convey my message because of limited attention spans. I watched the mothers' tired and distracted faces as I spoke about what a good attachment looks like and how it serves development. The mothers were thoughtful and attentive, absorbing what they could while focusing on their babies' needs.

I stopped after 15 minutes and asked if there were any questions. A mother with a baby snuggled against her looked at me and said, "What should I do to discipline him?" I was taken aback—what had her baby done to require discipline? My face must have conveyed surprise because she quickly added, "What I mean is how do I discipline him when he is older?" The truth is her question was not unlike many I'd had as a new mother or that I routinely hear from parents. The questions usually start the same way: "What should I do when my child does _____?" "What should I do when my child doesn't listen?" "What should I do when they won't go to sleep?" "What should I do when they hit their brother or sister?" Yet as I looked at this room bursting with new life, I was unsettled by her question. There was something more critical that I longed to be asked. I wanted her to ask me about the secrets for growth and the unlocking of human potential. I wanted to share with her the wonder of development and her role in it. Her question about discipline could be answered only by first considering how young children thrive and flourish. I wanted to take a step back from focusing on what to do in the moment and consider what she could do to create the conditions for healthy development. I wanted to focus on maturity as the ultimate answer to immaturity and how parenting is about patience, time, and good caretaking.

The message I wanted to convey isn't one new parents typically hear. I wanted to reveal that the secret to raising a child isn't about having all the answers but about *being* a child's answer. I wanted to share with them that parenting isn't something you can learn from a book, though books can help when you're trying to make sense of a child. I wanted to express that parenting isn't something you learn from your own parents, though great ones are wonderful templates. I wanted to reaffirm that caring for a child knows no gender, age, or ethnicity. I wanted to reassure them that their feelings of responsibility, guilt, alarm, and caring were the instinctive and emotional underpinnings of becoming the parent their child needs. I wanted to convey that what every child requires is a place of rest so that they can play and grow. This doesn't require perfection from a parent, or knowing what to do all the time. What it requires is a yearning to be their child's best bet and to work at creating the conditions to foster their growth.

Becoming a Child's Best Bet

YOUNG CHILDREN ARE some of the most loved people around, but they are also some of the most misunderstood. Their unique personalities can be challenging for adults, as they routinely defy logic and understanding. They can act brazen, noncompliant, and defiant one minute, only to turn around and light up a room with their infectious giggles and joy. Given the unpredictable nature of young children, it is understandable why parents long for techniques and tools to deal with their immature behaviour. The problem is, instructions won't help a parent make sense of a child.

Becoming a child's best bet requires understanding them from the inside out. It requires insight, not skill. It is more about what we see when we look at our child than it is about what we do. It is about being able to hold on to the big developmental picture instead of getting lost in the details of daily living. Simply put, perspective is everything. If we see a young child as being in distress, we may seek to comfort them, but if we see a child as being manipulative, we may back away. If we see a young child as being defiant, we may move to punish them, but if we understand that children have instincts to resist, we can find a way through the impasse. If we see a young child as being too emotional, we may try to calm them down, but if we understand that strong emotions need to be expressed, we will help them learn a language of the heart. If we see a young child who cannot focus as having a disordered brain, we may medicate them, but if we see them as being immature, we may give them some time to grow up.

When we make sense of a child—when we start to understand the developmental reasons for their actions—their aggression can feel less personal, their opposition less provocative, and our focus can turn to creating the conditions that foster growth. It is hard to make headway with behaviour when we don't understand what is driving it, or when our own emotions cloud the picture. Charlie, a father of two young children, said, "I used to be the most laid-back person around. You could ask any of my friends and they'd say I was the most easygoing out of all of them. Now that I have children, I think I have an anger management problem." Similarly, Samantha, a mother of two young boys, wrote, "I have come to realize my kids aren't trying to grate on my single last nerve and I have started to enjoy them again." The bottom line is, our reactions to young children are based upon what we see, which ultimately informs what we do. Most importantly, what we do informs our child about the type of care they can expect from us.

Young children represent immaturity at its best and illuminate the raw beginnings from which we grow. Although we may watch their immature ways in horror, we may also be filled with awe and wonder as human life renews itself again. The secret to unlocking the ancient patterns of human growth lies not in *what we do* to our young children but in *who we are* to them. Within our children is the promise of a mature future we play midwife to—and this is why making sense of them matters.

The Neufeld Approach

REST, PLAY, GROW is grounded in the integrated, attachment-based, and developmental approach to making sense of kids created by Gordon Neufeld. Neufeld is an internationally acclaimed and respected developmental psychologist whose work has been the creation of a coherent, cohesive, comprehensive theoretical model of human development. Neufeld has put the pieces of the developmental puzzle together based on more than 40 years of research, as well as practice. His theoretical model is drawn from many disciplines, including neuroscience, developmental psychology, attachment science, depth psychology, and cultural tradition. It provides a road map to understanding how human maturation unfolds from birth to adulthood as well as the failure to psychologically mature. Strategies for intervening with children are neither contrived nor divorced from natural development or human relationships. At the centre of the Neufeld approach is the primary developmental agenda of making sense of the conditions required for the realization of human potential. The goal is to put adults back into the driver's seat by making sense of a child from the inside out. In other words, a child's best bet is a parent who is the expert on that child.

My involvement with Gordon Neufeld began more than a decade ago, as a result of the many hats I wore: researcher, professor, counsellor, and, most importantly, parent. After decades of studying development, teaching students, and counselling clients, I encountered his work at a presentation on adolescence. Within the first hour, I was captivated by how he had made sense of my own adolescence and explained the behaviour of so many of the students I taught and counselled. His work became transformational in my understanding of human development, especially vulnerability, attachment, and maturation. I realized that my focus had become too narrow, as I considered behaviour without making sense of growth. I was working with people diagnosed with disorders without fully understanding human vulnerability. I was offering treatment and giving advice for problems I needed to make sense of at the root. I had become, without knowing it, lost in research results and practices divorced from insight, with no way to put the pieces of the puzzle together. Listening to Gordon Neufeld returned me to common sense and put insight at the fore again.

It was not long after this that I began immersing myself in earnest in the study of human maturation, attachment, and vulnerability through the Neufeld Institute. Two years later, I sat across from Gordon on his patio on a beautiful spring evening as he interviewed me for a postdoctoral internship with him. I had asked him prior to the meeting if there was anything I needed to do to prepare, and he'd told me, "No, what is needed is already inside of you. Just show up." His questions that evening were deceptively simple but sought understanding of why I wished to study with him. I told him the theory he had constructed had brought the human condition into focus for me; I was more effective as a counsellor in getting to root issues and in building relationships with students, and it had transformed my parenting. I told him I felt compelled to ensure that his work never got lost and that I wished to help parents and professionals make sense of kids. He obviously liked my answer because

I am still here more than ten years later, writing about all I have learned.

The theoretical content and images throughout *Rest, Play, Grow* are used with permission of Gordon Neufeld and are based on course material created by him. This material spans more than 14 courses offered through the Neufeld Institute, totalling over 100 hours of instruction. I am grateful for his permission to generously borrow and follow on his pioneering work as a theorist and teacher. For further information on the Neufeld Institute and its courses, please see the back of this book.

Although *Rest, Play, Grow* is based on Neufeld's theory, it is illustrated from my own experiences as a parent and professional. It is the book I wish I'd had when my children were younger, and the one I hope to give them when they become parents. It is based on stories about young children shared with me by parents, teachers, child care providers, Neufeld parent educators and faculty, and health care professionals, and on my own experiences as a mother. My approach as a researcher and writer has always been qualitative, bringing a phenomenon to life with rich examples to increase insight and understanding. I have shared the material on young children here through this lens to make it relevant to adults, to foster insight, and to help make sense of the child who is right in front of you. All of the identifying information has been changed, so any resemblance to real people is purely coincidental. The one exception is Gail's story in chapter 3. Gail was a cherished faculty member at the Neufeld Institute who loved to teach about play and young children.

What Does It Mean to Rest, Play, Grow?

THE PHRASE "Rest, Play, Grow" represents a developmental road map that paves the way for understanding how children reach their full human potential. This potential is not about academic achievements, social status or good behaviour, individual talents or gifts.

The developmental road map is about leading a child to maturity, to responsible citizenship, and to considering the world around them from multiple perspectives. It is a road map for growing a child into a separate, independent being who assumes responsibility for directing their own life and for the choices they make. It is about the unfolding of a child's potential as an adaptive being with the capacity to overcome adversity, persist in the face of difficulty, and become resilient. It is a road map to a child's potential as a social being who shares thoughts and feelings in a responsible way; develops impulse control, patience, and consideration; and considers the impact of who they are on others. It is a road map to guide what parents, teachers, child care providers, grandparents, aunts and uncles—any adult with a significant role—do so that a child can develop as a whole person. It lays out how an adult must WORK so that children can REST, so that they can PLAY and then GROW.

Rest, Play, Grow is meant to provide depth and breadth in understanding the young child while pointing to how adults create the conditions for healthy development. Although each chapter is distinct in focus, together they bring the young child into view and reveal how growth is the ultimate answer to underlying immaturity. Rest, Play, Grow discusses how play is critical to a child's development, how attachment provides the context in which to foster rest and raise a child, how emotions are the engine that drives growth, and how to deal with issues such as tears, tantrums, anxiety, separation, resistance, defiance, and, of course, discipline. The final chapter discusses how parents grow as a result of raising a child; I hope it alleviates concerns that you have to be fully mature before you become a parent.

This book is not about tips, techniques, mantras, instructions, or directions, though strategies are provided to help parents find their own way based on personal insight. It reaffirms parenting intuition and common sense, and brings comfort that you are not the only person who is baffled by your young child. It offers clarity where there is confusion, perspective where there is frustration, and patience knowing there is a natural developmental plan to grow a young child up. It is a book about taking care of young children as they are—egocentric, impulsive, inconsiderate, delightful, curious, joyful. It is about realizing that their immaturity isn't a mistake but the humble beginning from which we all start. *Rest, Play, Grow* is about using insight to make sense of a child, having confidence in what you see, and having faith to take care of them from that place inside of you. Although this book is a road map for parents who want to be their child's best bet, it is also what every young child wishes their adults understood about them.

How Adults Grow
Young Children Up

Understanding is love's other name.
If you don't understand, you can't love.
—THÍCH NHẤT HẠNH[1]

THE BEST PLACE to witness the spectacle of early childhood is the playground. Young children burst forth full of life, with legs running, arms waving, and torsos twisting down slides. Budding scientists are left to their own devices as they explore puddles and stare at worms. Their clothing reflects their internal energy: vibrant colours and patterns spring to life on moving bodies. Some speak a different language, one of lost words and dropped or altered consonants, from "ret's go to da swide" to "I wan somefing eat." You can't help but grin at the toddlers (aptly named for their wobbly legs) moving their top-heavy bodies through space while learning about gravity. On a sunny day the playground buzzes vibrantly, reverberating energy throughout adjacent neighbourhoods. There are snacks galore, and greedy crows perch on rooftops waiting to feast when opportunity arises. Adults share ideas about fussy eaters and troubled sleepers, home and work balance, and strategies for dealing with tantrums. There is a palpable hunger in the adults to make sense of their young children and connect with mature people.

All of a sudden the air is pierced by a child's fire-drill scream protesting their parent's desire to leave: "Noooooo... I don't wanna goooo!" The adults share sympathetic nods while secretly delighting that it isn't their child having a meltdown. A child runs off immune to his parent's directions, while another defiantly declares, "I do it myself!" Two boys wrestle over a bucket declaring "It's mine" and "I want it!" Suddenly, a desperate voice screams, "I have to go poo," launching her caregiver into action. A tired parent runs off to help a toddler who has fallen over and is crying in frustration.

Here, in this fenced-off world of red, yellow, and blue play equipment, lies a developmental snapshot of the splendour, wonder, and challenges of raising young children. In these small bodies exist the potential for growth and the promise of a mature future. The chasm between their immaturity and future maturity feels enormous. They are inconsiderate, impulsive, curious, and self-absorbed little people. Young children don't think like us, talk like us, or act like us, but care for them we must.

The Wonder of Development

AS A CHILD, I felt a sense of awe and wonder watching bean seeds unfold in water-laden, paper-towel-stuffed jars. The mythical beanstalks would stretch towards the light, breaking free from their seed casings. How did a seed contain the blueprint for its own development and burst forth to reveal a new life form?

My grandfather would often tour me through his vegetable garden, indulging my curiosity and my fascination with the natural world. As a master gardener, he was amused at my impatience at having to wait for things to grow. He tutored me on how to tend to the soil, on the specific conditions each plant required, and on how to keep a watchful eye. As he shared the bounty of his garden, I felt an unspoken gratefulness for his diligent caretaking. I know he would have taken great delight in watching my children dig up potatoes as if they were buried treasure.

Today my wonder and fascination have turned to how young children grow. The transformation that occurs in the early years is nothing short of magical. Children are launched from their watery existence without the full capacity for vision, language, or mobility. Over time they learn to walk and talk, and take steps towards interacting with people and things. Like little scientists they explore and take samples from their environment, experiencing the mundane as a new discovery. They have an unparalleled spirit and appetite for learning. Their desire to make sense of the world lacks concern over what they do not know. True to their developmental potential, they grow right under our noses while we track height measurements on the wall.

The thing I cherish most about young children is how immaturity influences the world they see. They operate with incomplete information and are unable to grasp the big picture. I watched a preschooler point at a police officer's handcuffs and ask, "Are those your coffee holders?" Another child wanted to know why an officer would use a police baton to smash a car window to open a door instead of "just using the door handle like we do." Young children are in the midst of putting the world together one piece at a time, and their questions reveal the newly discovered parts. A four-year-old boy declared to his mother, "Ham comes from pigs because they are both pink." He was also confident that "when pigs get old, they just walk and walk until the ham falls off." Young children see a world that is not constrained by adult logic.

Through scientific endeavours, we try to make sense of young children, from unravelling brain and emotional development to fostering their self-control. These discoveries are remarkable, but I am captivated by what science cannot explain. How can we measure young children's delight, frustration, and wonder as they learn about their world? I used to watch my children become mesmerized by dust particles glittering in the sunlight after opening window blinds. Even as household cleanliness loomed in my head, I wondered how they could render dust so delightful. While we act as children's guides in a foreign land, they translate the world back to us. With fresh eyes they reveal the things we have grown accustomed to or have missed. From the fascination of discovering a ladybug to the delicious taste of ice cream, the simple things are made sweeter. Young children live in the moment, and if we follow them, they take us there too.

Young children are curious and remarkable beings, so the question of how we grow them up can feel both daunting and fascinating. For thousands of years we have raised them according to cultural tradition and in keeping with the context we find ourselves in. Families and communities have rooted children, providing them with answers to key questions: Who am I? Where do I come from? Where do I belong? As we assume responsibility for taking care of children, we are faced with considering how they develop in the first place. What are the necessary conditions to support healthy growth?

Parents find there is no shortage of advice on the *physical needs* of young children. We keep a watchful eye on their health, diet, and fitness while their limbs silently grow longer. We measure height, weight, temperature, and movement to determine if we are on track. When they are sick, we take care of them, trusting that their body has defences to help with their healing too. We seem to trust intuitively in the developmental potentials that have guided physical growth for centuries, knowing that our role is to provide the conditions for well-being.

A child also develops *psychologically*, growing towards personhood and separate functioning, with innate inner potentials also guiding this. Just as in physical development, growth is not assured unless the right conditions have been provided. Information and advice are readily available on the emotional and social well-being of children, but this material is often overwhelming and confusing. Advice varies depending on which expert you speak to, with sound bites and other fragments disconnected from developmental science. Natural parenting insight and intuition have been diminished in favour of increasing reliance on others to provide instructions on how to raise children.

The literature on raising psychologically healthy children is further complicated by competing and contradictory perspectives. The prevailing behavioural/learning paradigm exists in stark contrast to the developmental/relational model. The bulk of parenting techniques and practices today are based on behavioural views of human nature, supported by professionals trained in this approach. At the core of behaviourism is an underlying belief that it is *unnecessary* to understand emotion or intentions to make sense of or change someone's behaviour.[2] B.F. Skinner, a psychologist and leading proponent of the behavioural approach, considered emotions to be private and inaccessible. He focused on behaviour that could be controlled and measured. Emotions were seen as nuisance variables, as byproducts of behaviour but never as the underlying cause of it.[3]

In a behavioural/learning approach, a child's behaviour is shaped and maturity is taught. The unspoken assumption is that a child learns to be mature, with parents controlling this process rather than growing them towards maturity by providing the conditions for it to unfold. The father of behaviourism, John B. Watson, said, "Give me a dozen healthy infants, well-formed, and my own specified world to bring them up in and I'll guarantee to take any one at random and train him to become any type of specialist I might select—doctor, lawyer, artist, merchant-chief and, yes, even beggar-man and thief, regardless of his talents, penchants, tendencies, abilities, vocations, and race of his ancestors."[4] The legacy of these words has been a proliferation of child-rearing practices that rely on sculpting techniques, such as negative or positive reinforcement, rewards, consequences, and coercion, to correct signs of immaturity. Dealing with a child's immature behaviour is the primary focus, and parenting skills are used to modify learned responses. In this approach, emotions are largely ignored and are believed to fall into line once behaviour and thinking are fixed.

Fortunately, the behavioural worldview is under scrutiny and faces increasing challenge given the mounting neuroscientific evidence of the pivotal role of human attachment and emotion in healthy development.[5] It is now accepted by leading neuroscientists that the human brain comes prewired with a motivational system made up of impulses, instincts, and emotions that are innate, not learned.[6] The goal in raising a child is to bring emotions, instincts, and impulses under a system of intention giving rise to civilized behaviour. The innate forces that were once ignored in a behavioural approach have now come into the fore and are viewed as pivotal in shaping the brain and human potential.

In the developmental/relational approach, parents are like gardeners who seek to understand what conditions children grow best in. Their focus is on cultivating strong adult–child relationships that provide the foundation on which full human potential is realized. Parents use their relationship to protect and preserve a child's emotional functioning and well-being. Developmentalists don't seek to carve maturity into a child but work to support the conditions to grow children up organically. There is a natural development plan that drives growth, and parents are the key providers when it comes to creating the conditions to unlock it. Just as in physical growth, children are born with inner growth processes that, if supported, propel them towards greater psychological and emotional maturity. Maturation is spontaneous but not inevitable. Children are like seeds: they need the right warmth, nourishment, and protection to grow.

What young children need most of all is at least one adult who can satiate their hunger for contact and closeness. Urie Bronfenbenner, the founder of the Head Start Program, said, "Every child needs at least one adult who is irrationally crazy about him or her."[7] The womb of personhood is a relational one. More than 60 years of attachment research, from psychology to neuroscience, have converged on the importance of the parent–child relationship in healthy growth and development.[8] As John Bowlby said to the World Health Organization in Geneva, "What is believed to be essential for mental health is that the infant and young child should experience a warm, intimate and continuous relationship with his mother (or permanent mother-substitute) in which both find satisfaction and enjoyment."[9]

When children's relational needs are satiated, they will be freed from their greatest hunger and at rest—released to their play. It is in play that they grow and morph into the chefs, engineers, carpenters, teachers, or astronauts of tomorrow. It is on the relational playgrounds we create for them that they will discover their true form, free of any consequences that would bind them to permanence. It is in our gardens that they must feel free to express what is within their hearts without fear of repercussion to our relationship, and where the person they become slowly takes shape, free of pressure and the need for performance. A garden of growth can be cultivated only by generously offering children fulfilling relationships to tether themselves to. If you are not rooted, you cannot grow. When we take care of our children's relational needs and ensure that their hearts are soft, nature will take care of the rest. We need to work not at growing our children up but at cultivating the relational gardens in which they flourish.

Human development is a wondrous and remarkable thing. Through our young children we are afforded glimpses into how we humans grow into separate beings and the changes that occur along the way. The good news is, nature has a blueprint to grow children up, not only physically but psychologically as well. As we create the conditions for their growth, we play midwife to the developmental potential that resides in them. The challenge is that our caretaking gaze needs to be focused on the antecedents that support growth, just as my grandfather focused when he tended the soil and understood what each plant needed to thrive. Nature was not ill intended in giving us such impulsive, inconsiderate, and egocentric beings—there was a method to the madness, a plan to be unfolded. We have become impatient when it comes to psychological development. We have become sculptors instead of the master gardeners our young children require. This stems not from a lack of caring about our children but from a lack of understanding as to how maturity unfolds.

The Three Maturation Processes*

WHAT DOES IT mean to raise a child to reach their full human potential and how will we know we are there? Parents are fairly uniform in the characteristics they desire in children. When asked what is most important to them, 93 percent of parents want their child to become independent and take responsibility for their life. Secondary were values of hard work, helping others, creativity, empathy, tolerance, and persistence.[10] Parents know the end goal but are unsure how maturity is achieved given their child's uncivilized beginnings. What are the inner growth processes that drive a child to become a socially and emotionally responsible individual?

Based on decades of distilling developmental research, theory, and practice to the essence, Gordon Neufeld has put the pieces together to form a coherent theory of human maturation. Growth is driven by three distinct inner processes, which are spontaneous in development but not inevitable: (1) The emergent process gives rise to the capacity to function as a *separate person* and to develop a strong sense of agency. (2) The adaptive process enables a person to *adapt* to life circumstances and overcome adversity. (3) The integrative process helps a child grow into a *social being* with the capacity to engage in relationships without compromising personal integrity and identity. The presence or absence of the emergent, adaptive, and

---

* From Gordon Neufeld, "Synthesis of the Unfolding of Human Potential," *Neufeld Intensive I: Making Sense of Kids*, course (Neufeld Institute, Vancouver, BC, 2013).

integrative processes are the measurements or "vital signs" we can use to assess the developmental trajectory of a child and their overall maturity. It is our human potential to become *separate, adaptive, and social beings*, but this can be realized only when adults play a supportive role in cultivating the conditions for growth.[11]

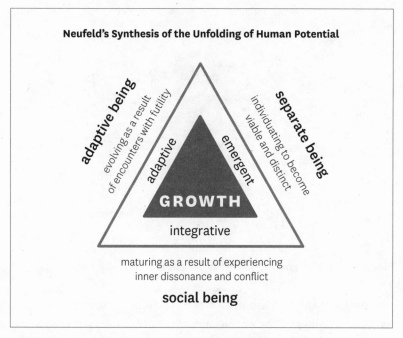

Neufeld's Synthesis of the Unfolding of Human Potential

adaptive being

evolving as a result of encounters with futility

separate being

individuating to become viable and distinct

adaptive

emergent

GROWTH

integrative

maturing as a result of experiencing inner dissonance and conflict

social being

Figure 1.1 Taken from *Neufeld Intensive I: Making Sense of Kids* course

The first goal of healthy development is viability as a *separate being* and involves gradual movement from dependence to independence to adult autonomy through the *emergent process*. The emergent process thrusts a child towards selfhood and exploration of their world. Play is the natural sphere in which children first start to express this emergent self, the birthplace of growth into personhood, but it only occurs when children are at rest in relationships with caring adults.

The emergent process bears many fruits, including a capacity to function when separate from one's attachments as well as to form interests and goals. Emergent children exude a wonderful vitality and are rarely bored. There is vibrancy to life, a sense of wonder, and a curiosity that leads to experimentation, imagining, and daydreaming. It is through this emergent process that imaginary friends are born.

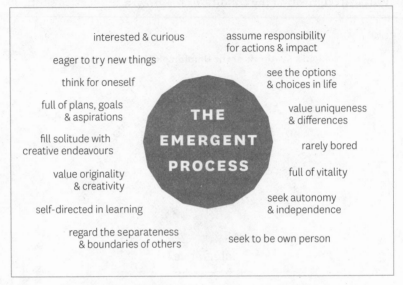

interested & curious

eager to try new things

think for oneself

full of plans, goals
& aspirations

fill solitude with
creative endeavours

value originality
& creativity

self-directed in learning

regard the separateness
& boundaries of others

assume responsibility
for actions & impact

see the options
& choices in life

value uniqueness
& differences

rarely bored

full of vitality

seek autonomy
& independence

seek to be own person

THE EMERGENT PROCESS

Figure 1.2 Taken from *Neufeld Intensive I: Making Sense of Kids* course

Emergent children are also known for their venturing forth spirit, which drives them to be enthusiastic learners as they strive to make sense of the world. They actively shape and assume responsibility for their life story instead of becoming a character in someone else's. There is such a strong desire to be a unique being that plagiarizing, copying, or imitating are rejected as affronts to the integrity of self-hood. The anthem of an emergent child is "Me-do" or "I do it myself." Dealing with the natural resistance and opposition that arrive to make room for selfhood is addressed in chapter 9.

The second maturation process that underlies human potential is the *adaptive process*. It is at the root of how we become resilient and resourceful, and how we recover from adversity. You cannot teach a child to become adaptive, and this process is not realized without the right conditions being present. The adaptive process helps equip children with the resilience to handle what lies ahead and thrive despite obstacles. It enables children to learn from mistakes, benefit from correction, and engage in trial and error. The adaptive process underlies our capacity to transform when up against things in our world we cannot change.

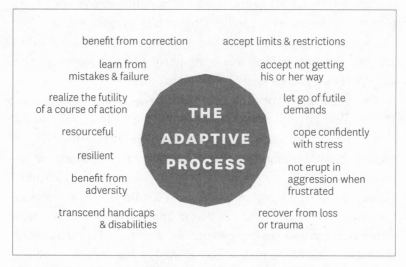

benefit from correction

learn from
mistakes & failure

realize the futility
of a course of action

resourceful

resilient

benefit from
adversity

transcend handicaps
& disabilities

THE ADAPTIVE PROCESS

accept limits & restrictions

accept not getting
his or her way

let go of futile
demands

cope confidently
with stress

not erupt in
aggression when
frustrated

recover from loss
or trauma

Figure 1.3 Taken from *Neufeld Intensive I: Making Sense of Kids* course

The adaptive process is also the answer to dealing with tantrums and aggression in young children (more about this in chapter 7). They are routinely upset when their agendas are thwarted, unleashing frustration and attempts to negotiate a better outcome. They are not born preprogrammed with a set of limits and restrictions that prepare them for everyday life. They sometimes look at us in amazement as if to say, "Why can't I have another cookie? What kind of place is this?!"

Young children are driven to possess, be first, and get what they want because of their egocentric nature. The adaptive process helps them relinquish their agendas and realize they can survive when things don't go their way. One of the fastest ways to create an "entitled" or "spoiled" child is to circumvent the adaptive process and prevent feelings of upset from occurring about all the things they cannot change. The character Veruca Salt in Willy Wonka and the Chocolate Factory is the epitome of such a child. She orders her parents around continually: "I want it, and I want it now, Daddy!" The parents live in fear of her eruptions and busy themselves constantly meeting her demands. A parent's job is to help prepare a child to live in the world as it exists, with the upsets and disappointments that are part of it. Parents' key role in supporting a child's growth as an adaptive being is discussed further in chapter 7.

The third maturation process that grows a child is integration. This process is responsible for transforming children into social beings who are mature and responsible. The integrative process requires brain development and emotional maturity. Based on the work of Jean Piaget, the phrase "5-to-7 shift" was coined by Sheldon White, signalling a significant change in cognitive development in a young child. At this time a child can appreciate context and take into account more than one perspective at a time.[12] This shift marks the natural end to the preschooler mentality and ushers in the age of reason and responsibility.[13] As this shift occurs, young children will become increasingly tempered in their expression of thoughts and feelings. They will start to exhibit impulse control in the face of strong emotions. Instead of lashing out, they might say, "I half hate you right now!" and "I want to hit you!" but they do not. They will exhibit patience, despite frustration at having to wait. They will be capable of sharing from a place of true consideration and not because they are told to do so. They will be able to persist towards a goal without collapsing in frustration. A civilized form will slowly appear and naturally diminish the immature ways of relating known as "the preschooler personality," discussed in chapter 2.

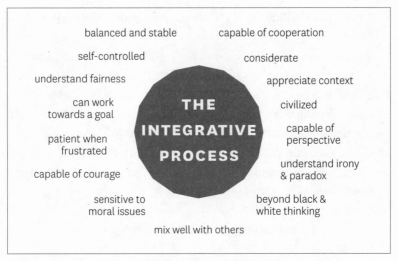

balanced and stable   capable of cooperation

self-controlled   considerate

understand fairness   appreciate context

can work   **THE**   civilized
towards a goal
                  INTEGRATIVE
                                         capable of
patient when   **PROCESS**   perspective
frustrated
                                         understand irony
capable of courage   & paradox

sensitive to   beyond black &
moral issues   white thinking

mix well with others

Figure 1.4 Taken from *Neufeld Intensive I: Making Sense of Kids* course

One of the most important developmental resolutions of the integrative process is the capacity to be a separate self in the midst of so many other people. When you are able to hold on to your own point of view while considering another person's experiences, it provides greater breadth and depth in perspective. Young children can operate out of only one perspective at a time, and it is usually expressed as "It's mine." A mature person should be able to disagree with someone while preserving a sense of togetherness: "I can see your point of view—would you like to hear mine?" Integration should also give rise to a separate self that doesn't succumb to peer pressure, blending, cloning, or fusing. As Katie, a seven-year-old girl, said to her friend while playing, "I don't want to be your pet baby rabbit. I don't like rabbits. I want to be the hamster mother instead."

Our ultimate destiny as social beings is to fully participate in our communities and possess a level of moral reasoning that goes beyond the "I" and considers the needs of the whole. If we want our children to participate as global citizens and become stewards of the earth, they need to become mature social beings. Our potential as social beings is unlocked through healthy parent–child relationships.

There is an organic solution to the immaturity of young children. There is a natural developmental process, and parents have a critical role in it. When the conditions for growth have been assured, the inner emergent, adaptive, and integration processes will launch a child's trajectory towards personhood. A failure to mature is also part of the human condition, but this is where adults must be a child's best bet. Selfhood cannot be taught or forced; it must be nurtured, cultivated, preserved, and protected.

Preserving the Spirit of Childhood

WHILE PRESENTING TO a parent group one evening, I overheard a mother read the title of Gordon Neufeld and Gabor Maté's book, *Hold On to Your Kids*.[14] With an alarmed voice she turned to her friend and said, "Hold on to your kids? Seriously? Where's the book that tells you how to get rid of them?!" This sentiment captures the hurry we seem to be in to get our children to grow up and act mature. It seems we have lost patience with immaturity and believe our children can be harvested sooner. In moments of desperation and frustration, we may resort to demanding of a child, "Just grow up!" Alas, we cannot speed up, command, demand, prod, push, pull, bribe, threaten, reward, cajole, or give children a pill to grow up.

When it comes to young children, there is no disagreement about whether maturity is desired, but there are substantial differences in ideas of *how to get there*. Do we grow children, or do we try to control development? If we are in a hurry, we will push. If we believe that children should be given time and space to grow, we will create the conditions for natural development to unfold. We cannot do both. Good development requires patience and faith. The problem with pushing and controlling is they can interfere with providing what children really need. They can create stressful environments where children feel there is something wrong with the way they are. When young children are pushed towards independence too quickly, it can make them cling to us out of insecurity. In our pursuit to have them take on a mature form earlier than nature intended, we can diminish, confine, and crush the spirit of childhood. Yet our pushing continues despite decades of developmental science demonstrating that the principles governing growth do not change.

One of the biggest challenges for parents today is in preserving the spirit of childhood. The word *spirit* stems from the Latin word for "breath" or "vigour." Spirit is what underlies children's vitality and their propensity to grow, to unfold, and to become. When we are consumed with the mature form our children take without preserving their spirit, the results can be short-lived and superficial. There is a difference between the child who *acts* mature and the child who is given time to *become* mature. We have become distracted, confused, and lulled into believing that a mature performance is synonymous with maturity. We believe we can control growth instead of focusing on how we influence the conditions that give rise to it.

We can train a child to do a lot of things at early ages, but we shouldn't mistake this for maturity. The pediatrician T. Berry Brazelton wrote, "The human infant is amazingly capable of compliance. He can be shaped to walk at nine months, recite numbers at two, read by three, and he can even learn to cope with the pressures that lie behind these expectations. But children in our culture need someone who will cry out, 'At what price?' "[15] There are seasons to growth and forces that guide it. An apple seed looks nothing like the apple tree that bears fruit. When raised in a hurry, young children pay a price developmentally.

We want our children to emerge as socially and emotionally responsible individuals, but our society has become preoccupied with the caring performance given rather than the roots from which caring actions arise. For example, young children can be made to say "sorry" or "thank you," but this doesn't ensure that they feel remorse or gratitude. They even sense the insincerity in such actions, complaining to each other, "Say 'sorry' like you mean it!" When forced to say "sorry" or "thank you," their words are detached from the caring emotions that are meant to guide them. Any hurry to get a mature performance will thwart their understanding of the emotions that will render them the most humane. We cannot expect healthy moral development to unfold based on false fronts. Caring and compassionate children are homegrown by nurturing the emotional roots that sustain them. Becoming a social being starts with understanding oneself. The capacity to get along with others, show consideration, and take responsibility for one's actions are the results of healthy development. A child can be scripted to look civilized, but it is a performance devoid of any depth.

Further erosion of the spirit of childhood stems from the unspoken assumption that "earlier is better."[16] This ethos permeates expectations for behaviour and performance in the early years. David Elkind, a developmental psychologist and author of *Miseducation: Preschoolers at Risk*, says that in the 1970s parents hurried their children, in the 1980s they wanted superkids, and in the 1990s they wanted to give their child a competitive advantage over others.[17] At the turn of the twenty-first century, early childhood is still under threat as it becomes reengineered to accelerate growth.

Part of the problem is that many parents have lost faith, have become disoriented, and are culturally adrift from a developmental view of human nature. What has happened to our inherent faith that children will grow with time, patience, and care? The rapid social, economic, and technological changes of the last 100 years have dismantled cultural wisdom regarding children and how they grow. Guiding beliefs in acceleration and performance continue to infiltrate and pressurize early childhood. Hundreds of years of parenting tradition are now fragmented and without cultural moorings. We are no longer clear what future we are preparing our children for.[18] Most parents today are digital immigrants raising children who are the first true digital natives of the Information Age.[19]

The shift from agricultural to industrial to information societies over the last 100-plus years has meant we are less governed by the natural rhythms that have sustained life for centuries.[20] In a digital world, we no longer live our lives in accordance with the cycles of the moon, the sun, and the seasons. The rhythms of the natural world are now displaced by timing that is 24/7 and global. Steve Jobs is quoted as saying he "never liked to put on-off switches on Apple devices."[21] Although our new tools and devices promise to deliver us neverending services, increased performance, and connectivity, they run counter to the developmental principles and futilities that govern human life. Our new tools and technologies are detaching us from the steady hum of life's natural rhythms. We can do many things faster, but raising children wasn't meant to be one of them.

The question we need to ask ourselves is what is our role in growing a child up? A parent is a key provider in a child's life, critical to creating the conditions for growth and for protecting the spirit of childhood. We must start with asking the right questions to guide us, the ones that are concerned with how children thrive, flourish, and become their own person. The answer to immaturity is maturity, which unfolds when adults become the answer to a child's relational and emotional needs. Parents play midwife to the promise of human potential that resides in each child. To do this we need to become conscious of our role in nature's plan so as to counter and buffer against today's social upheaval amid global technological transformation. We are fortunate to have developmental science to guide us, to help validate parenting intuition, to support cultural traditions in raising children, and to provide insight when we feel lost. Master gardeners use science and intuition to know what is needed for good growth and have faith that potential arises from cultivating deep roots to tether all life.

2

The Preschooler Personality
Part Beauty, Part Beast

I could well envy you
Because you have no inkling of these troubles:
The happiest life consists in ignorance,
Before you learn to grieve and to rejoice.
SOPHOCLES[1]

YOUNG CHILDREN DON'T multitask, think twice, or say things like "Part of me feels like throwing a train at your head, while the other side of me thinks I should use my words instead." They don't *contemplate* their feelings; they *embody* their feelings, and are moved to attack or react impulsively. They are anything but predictable, with hurricane-force winds hurling them from one emotion, thought, or behaviour to the next. They experience the world in a singular fashion—one thought or feeling at a time—so everything is a big deal to them. They will be on or off, up or down, hot or cold, good or bad, this or that, but never in between. Young children aren't known for being moderate, fair, reasonable, considerate, thoughtful, or attentive. They know much better than they behave, and their good intentions seem to be short-lived.

Young children lack the capacity to consider more than one point of view at a time because their brains are still under development.

28

They are either Beauty or Beast, which doesn't bother them because they lack internal conflict and a developed conscience. Young children have an unparalleled capacity to defy logic and baffle their caretakers, as the following conversation with a parent of a preschooler exemplifies:

Mother: My three-year-old son just had a meltdown, screaming at the top of his lungs, crying, throwing, stomping, and pushing us away. He was really scaring his baby sister—and us too. I have never seen anything like this before! We tried to comfort him, but nothing worked. My husband got his blanket, and as soon as he gave it to him, he snuggled into it, started singing, and was happy! My husband and I are worried. Do you think he has a mental health problem? What is going on with him?

Deborah: Your son operates out of a preschooler personality, which is natural given he is three years old. He can only do one emotion or thought at a time, so when you gave him the blanket, his frustration was eclipsed by joy. He doesn't have a mental health problem. Your son is just immature. In fact, if you wanted to study human emotions, young children are the best subjects, as they experience them in such a pure form, untempered by any other experience.

Mother: What am I supposed to do then? How am I supposed to grow him out of this?

Deborah: Love, patience, time, good caretaking by you and your husband. Even in the face of these emotional expressions, you need to preserve your relationship and help him express and name his feelings whenever you can. Eventually, hits and stomps should become words of frustration, and he should naturally show signs of tempering, self-control, and consideration between the ages of 5 and 7 if all is unfolding well.

Mother: (Gasps) Seriously? We have to wait that long? Why didn't anyone tell us this? What am I going to tell my husband?

Deborah: That your one-year-old has the same thing, and there is nothing like the force of an immature child to test the maturity level in a parent.

The Preschooler Brain

. . . .

THE PRESCHOOLER PERSONALITY stems from brain immaturity and is characterized by behaviour that is obsessive, endearing, impulsive, anxious, delightful, unreflective, generous, unstable, aggressive, resistant, compulsive, and anything but predictable.[2] Young children experience a barrage of thoughts, feelings, impulses, and preferences but can't hold them together to form a clear picture. The "disorder" in the preschooler is not intentional but developmental. The role of adults is to create the conditions that will allow the brain to mature naturally and not to battle against symptoms of the preschooler personality.

Advances in neuroscience continue to map out how brain development unfolds in young children and how immature young children really are.[3] The brain is the most undifferentiated part of the body at birth, meaning its cells lack specific functioning and are open to being shaped by the environment, and development relies on contact and closeness with attachment figures to grow.[4] The first three years of life boast the most neural activity.[5] According to Daniel Siegel, a psychiatrist, neural pathways will grow rapidly, allowing neurons to communicate with each other with increasing speed, efficiency, and sophistication. Engagement with people and experiences will create, activate, or strengthen neural pathways. The brain is a living system, and the most sophisticated of any natural or artificial structure on Earth. It possesses the inherent capacity to reshape itself and adapt according to its environment.[6]

Young children's brains require, on average, five to seven years of healthy development to fully integrate; that is, for the parts of the brain to establish communication with each other. Brain integration is a global event that connects multiple layers of neural circuitry both vertically, starting at the base of the brain and working upwards, as well as bilaterally, with the left and right hemispheres connecting to each other over time.[7] The integration of right and left hemispheres in the prefrontal cortex is critical to the development of executive functions but takes longer than in other parts of the brain.[8] Executive functions include the capacity for judgement, flexible thinking, planning, organization, and self-control. They underpin the capacity for insight, imagination, creativity, problem solving, communication, empathy, morality, and wisdom. Until the prefrontal cortex is sufficiently integrated, a young child will remain impulsive and untempered.[9] Brain development continues into adolescence but changes significantly between 5 and 7 years of age.[10]

At the root of the preschooler personality is an immature brain that cannot make sense of all of the sensory input and signals it receives. Left and right hemispheres develop separately before they can communicate effectively with one another. As a result, a young child can attend to only one set of signals at a time. The brain purposely places a moratorium on contending with competing signals to allow the child to fully make sense of one thing at a time.

When young children become engrossed in something, they will become oblivious to the rest of the world. This is the brain's unique capacity to tune out competing stimuli in order to tune in on something. One day I watched a young child become entranced by a seashell at the beach. His brain worked hard to cut out conflicting stimuli in order to zero in on the shape, size, texture, and sound of the seashell. He was surprised and upset when he got splashed by a wave, as if it had snuck up on him. His lack of attention to his surroundings was not a mistake or sign of an attention problem but a strategic and purposeful design. Like blinders on a horse, his brain tuned out extraneous stimuli so that he could function, attend, and learn about a seashell in the midst of so much distraction.

When a child can sufficiently differentiate the signals from one another, the brain will integrate the signals in the prefrontal cortex with help from the corpus callosum.[11] In other words, the blinders come off and reveal the world in two dimensions because the cognitive apparatus is in place to make sense of conflicting signals.

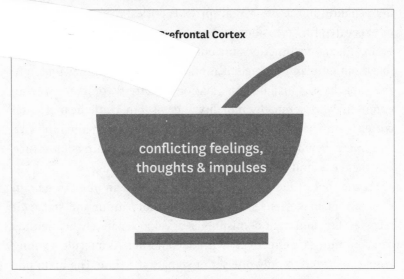

Prefrontal Cortex

conflicting feelings, thoughts & impulses

Figure 2.1 Adapted from *Neufeld Intensive I: Making Sense of Kids* course

When the right and left hemispheres are sufficiently developed, the prefrontal cortex will transform into a mixing bowl for conflicting feelings, thoughts, and impulses. This typically occurs between the ages of 5 and 7. A child will begin to experience inner dissonance and conscience will be born. For example, as a child goes to throw something in frustration, there may be a conflicting or competing impulse that says, "Don't throw, as you could hurt someone." Instead of their day being "good" or "bad," they might tell you it was both. They may report that they wanted to take something that wasn't theirs but stopped because they knew it was wrong. As a child enters the 5-to-7 shift, they are able to consider two aspects of a phenomenon at the same time and coordinate two different thoughts.[12]

It is the mixing of feelings and thoughts in the prefrontal cortex that ultimately puts the brakes on untempered acts and delivers self-control. Strong emotions and impulses find their antidote in competing strong emotions and impulses—they are meant to have a paralyzing effect when brought together. The internal conflict that is created by discordant feelings and thoughts brings emotional energy to a standstill. For example, the answer to *fear* is *desire*, which gives rise to *courage*. The answer to *frustration* is *caring*, which gives rise to *patience*. When feelings and thoughts are given enough space and encouraged to conflict, a wrestling match will ensue. The goal is to weave emotions and thoughts together, leading to a more mature temperament.

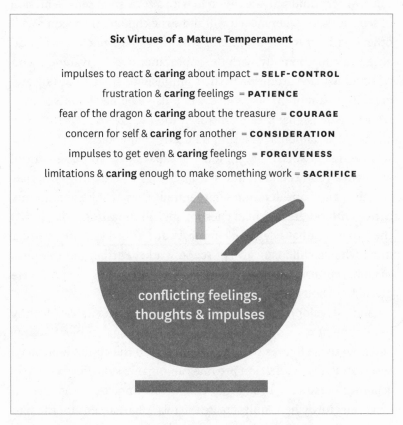

Six Virtues of a Mature Temperament

impulses to react & **caring** about impact = **SELF-CONTROL**
frustration & **caring** feelings = **PATIENCE**
fear of the dragon & **caring** about the treasure = **COURAGE**
concern for self & **caring** for another = **CONSIDERATION**
impulses to get even & **caring** feelings = **FORGIVENESS**
limitations & **caring** enough to make something work = **SACRIFICE**

conflicting feelings, thoughts & impulses

Figure 2.2 Taken from *Neufeld Intensive I: Making Sense of Kids* course

When the prefrontal cortex matures with hemispheric integration, the young child will transform as an individual and the preschooler days will come to a close. The importance of the 5-to-7 shift as a developmental milestone cannot be overstated. It is the ultimate answer to the preschooler personality and the birthplace of both personal and social integration.

With personal integration, the young child will be able to work towards achieving a goal, think before speaking, and restrain themselves when frustrated. They will appear more rational and reasonable, with more complex logical thinking. A coherent narrative can now form and provide the child with a consistent representation of self.[13] A more coherent self will allow the child to be together with others without losing a sense of who they are. The child will leap ahead developmentally, with the appearance of self-awareness, control, and focused attention.[14] Their impulsivity should subside and give rise to a more moderate, less impulsive being. Parents should rejoice at the signs of self-control in their child—one of the most critical developmental milestones in early childhood.

In terms of social integration, the capacity for impulse control will help a young child fit into social settings where turn taking, perspective, and consideration are required. They will be able to mix better with others and read cues for social interaction. Historically, the 5-to-7 shift has been used in most educational systems to determine when a child is ready for schoolwork.[15] Furthermore, studies of global cultural practices show that children at this age group are given more household responsibilities.[16]

Brain development is spontaneous but not inevitable. Healthy development rests on the availability of human attachment figures and how those figures become caretakers for the child's emotional system.[17] Brain maturation provides an organic solution to the preschooler personality but cannot be forced, practised, or pushed. Children grow when adults create the relational gardens for them to play and flourish in.

Sensitive or "Orchid" Children and Brain Integration

APPROXIMATELY ONE IN five children stands out as being more affected or stirred up than their peers by their environment.[18] They seem to be more easily overwhelmed, alarmed, intense, sensitive, and prickly in their responses, and passionate in temperament. Sensitive children have been called "orchid-like," compared with kids who grow with ease like dandelions.

Sensitive kids show greater receptivity and an enhanced capacity to take in their environment through the senses. It is like they have radio antennas that are tuned to maximum receptivity so as to avoid missing any signals. Although the type and level of receptivity differs from child to child, they will show heightened sensory responses in visual, auditory, touch, taste, smell, kinesthetic/proprioceptor (related to physical tension or chemical conditions within the body), and emotional/perceptual areas. The combinations are endless, and each child will present on a continuum of receptivity with each sense.

Sensitive children may complain that tags in their clothes are too itchy, sounds are too loud, smells are too strong, or some foods taste really bad. It can be difficult to get their attention because they are bombarded by sensory information and are overwhelmed. They also seem to possess a natural brightness in comparison to other children because of their enhanced receptivity to information and stimulation. Adults might see them as being overly dramatic or reactive, but they are only being true to the enormous world that exists inside them. A mother of a five-year-old sensitive boy was surprised by his reaction to a change in location for his music lesson and shared the following:

> Jacob loved his music teacher so much that when she had to change locations for her classes, we followed her from the sunlit classroom near our home to the dark basement music academy where she was

teaching. In the first class, Jacob couldn't settle in and kept running out the door. During the second class, he became so agitated he jumped up and down and landed on the teacher. A day later, when calm, I asked him if there was something about the new space that he didn't like. "The lights buzz," he explained. "I can't hear anything because of the lights."

Orchid children are more sensitive to child-rearing practices—they will either wither or thrive, depending on their environment.[19] When they are raised in stressful environments, they are more affected than their easygoing "dandelion" counterparts. They are more likely to suffer from mental health issues, addictions, and delinquency as a result of such conditions.[20] However, when sensitive children are raised under ideal conditions with the presence of caring adults, their development can surpass that of their dandelion counterparts: "An orchid child becomes a flower of unusual delicacy and beauty."[21] It is their *relational* environment that makes the developmental difference for them.

The sensitive child's heightened receptivity to their environment can lengthen brain integration by up to two years. Instead of the 5-to-7 shift, they may need one to two more years to mature depending on their sensitivity levels and environment. The additional time is used to create and integrate additional neural pathways to accommodate their increased sensory receptivity.[22] The goals are to provide conditions such that orchid children can rest in the care of their adults, to provide them enough room to play, and to preserve their emotional vulnerability in the face of distress.

One of the common mistakes made with sensitive children is to give them more sensory information because of their natural brightness. More is not better, and can trigger defences to shut out sensory information. They need time and space, with a lot of room to play, to process all the stimulation they experience.

Young Children in Action: One Thought or Feeling at a Time

ALTHOUGH WE UNDERSTAND that young children have brains that are still under development, this doesn't prevent us from setting expectations for behaviour that are out of sync with their capacity. Their Beauty-and-Beast-like nature shows up regularly and creates implications for how we care for them. The following are six themes arising from a young child's lack of personal and social integration.

1. **Young Children "Fill in the Blanks" When Making Sense of Their World**
   Young children are *unable to appreciate context or consider more than one element in solving a problem.* They see the world one part at a time, making them blind to many cues and pieces of contextual information that adults take for granted. They can't read context because they can't hold on to all the different perspectives at the same time. For example, a pregnant mother took her three-and-a-half-year-old to an ultrasound appointment to "get a look" at his sibling for the first time. He started to cry uncontrollably as he watched his sibling move across the screen. As his mother comforted him with "It's okay, the baby is all right, don't worry," the boy cried out, "No, Mommy, no! Why did you eat the baby?!" Parents and young children don't often share the same worldview, which can lead to many misunderstandings.

   Young children don't stop to consider all the details before proceeding. They are notorious for filling in the blanks whenever they need to. For example, when a mother asked her five-year-old son, Alex, how babies were made, after his kindergarten sex education class, she was shocked to hear, "Daddy puts a chicken inside of Mommy and it lays eggs." Young children are not bothered by their own ignorance because they can't see the gaps in their understanding. A father of a three-year-old boy said, "Stop biting your nails or all of the dirty bugs will go inside your mouth and make you sick." The child replied, "It's okay, Dad, I just spit out the bugs when I chew my fingers." Young children are literal and straightforward in translating the world around them, which is often as refreshing as it is amusing. As one child told her mother, "When I was little I thought 'jersey cows' wore hockey jerseys. I was really surprised when I found out they didn't."

2. Young Children Tell It Like It Is and Know Much Better Than They Behave

Young children are *untempered in expression and experience, with no self-control*. They don't pause to think before they act; they just move according to instinct and emotion. Political or social correctness doesn't exist in their mindset, and they will share their ideas freely. A kindergartner was asked to draw a picture of his biggest accomplishment for his teacher. She asked him to explain, and he said, "This is me surviving my birth. This is my mom's 'bagina' and my head coming out." Young children are renowned for revealing family details, such as "Grandma, you have short legs," or "I have to take a nap so Mommy can have sanity time." Even with houseguests, young children don't think twice about yelling, "Wipe my bum!" or telling visitors, "I don't like your present." The honesty of the young child is as heartening as it is embarrassing. One child asked her mother after taking one look at the dinner she had prepared, "Why do you always cook us food we won't like?"

The challenge is to preserve young children's integrity and not overreact or shame them for being true to themselves. If we are to invite our children to make sense of their world, we need to foster their tendency to report on it. With ideal development, young children will eventually think twice before speaking. Until this point, they need room to make sense of the world as it arises for them, though we can encourage this to be done in privacy with us.

Young children are not good at keeping secrets. This stems from their inability to attend to more than one thought at a time. Despite good intentions to keep something private, they "forget" in the moment because of overriding excitement. Similarly, young children are not able to tell a true lie, as they cannot hold on to truth and falsehood at the same time. With no back of the mind or internal conflict, they honestly believe what they tell you. A mother of a three-year-old said, "One day, I asked Eva if she knew how the fingerprint in my freshly cooked brownies had got there. With an innocent expression she said, 'I don't know?' despite the fact there were only two of us home. I waited five minutes and then asked, 'How did the brownies taste?' Eva looked at me and said, 'Oh, Mommy, they were delicious!' " It is ironic that lying represents a step towards maturity, but there is sophistication in being able to deflect people away from what you don't want them to see. It requires a capacity to think twice, to have perspective, and to consider context.

Young children can't help but act impulsively based on their instincts and feelings. They promise they will never hit again only to repeat the same offence within minutes. Young children see their impulses and actions as not being under their control or as separate from themselves. They can be just as surprised when their arms have hits or when their teeth want to bite. Matthias, a four-year-old boy, said to his mother, "How can my arms have hits for someone I love?" They often end up in altercations with other young children, with foul eruptions over turf and possessions. Their frustration often arises based on their own, personal form of expression, with good intentions eclipsed by strong emotions. Young children don't think; they react, are moved to attack, and are impulsive—this is the young child in action. The capacity for only one thought or feeling at a time underlies outbursts of frustration and aggression.

Young children's lack of internal conflict contributes not only to eruptions of frustration but to the escalation of fun as well. If a little splash was fun, then a bigger splash must be "funner." Unadulterated joy is the reason why the hugs of young children possess healing properties and their giggles are so infectious. Whoever captures their hearts is truly adored, as their delight contains no hidden agendas or unfinished business. Their hearts carry no bitterness, no unmet expectations, and no resentments. Their love is pure in its expression. One mother said, "Near the end of Great-Grandpa's life, he became quite frustrated with his failing body and trips to the hospital. One of his last true joys was spending time with his youngest great-grandchildren. Their innocent way of being in the world was the medicine he needed. Their hugs had a magical quality to them and improved his vital signs." Young children's experience of happiness is unfettered by the potential of loss. Ignorance can truly be blissful.

3. There Is No Middle Ground and Everything Is a Big Deal

Young children are *prone to displaced or pendulum-like reactions, and swing from one experience and emotion to the next.* There is no moderation or middle ground, and fairness is defined as having got what they wanted. They may act compliant one minute only to turn around and dig in their heels with resistance the next. Their worldviews are either black or white, with a clear absence of grey. Not only do young children swing from one emotion to the next, but they take their parents with them. In a study on parental life satisfaction, parents of young children had greater emotional swings from joy to frustration than their childless counterparts.[23]

As young children can experience only one emotion at a time, one feeling can displace another, creating confusion for their caretakers. For example, I watched a four-year-old boy who was upset with his mother when she told him he had to leave the beach. As his mother moved to comfort him, he hit her. She backed away and said, "No, Felix, you don't hit." Seeing the anger on his mother's face and her retreat, his frustration was quickly displaced by fear. He cried out in alarm, "Mama, Mama, Mama!" When the mother saw Felix's anguish, she rushed to his side again. As the reconnection was made, his alarm subsided only to be replaced by his residual frustration at having to leave the beach. He hit her again, and she backed away

5. It's All about Play and No Work

Young children are *unable to get the concept of work or to exhibit goal-directed behaviour where sacrifice is required*. This tends to worry many parents who view perseverance and sacrifice to be at the heart of success in life, from sports and hobbies to school and work. They are exasperated at their young child's shortsightedness and perceived lack of motivation, their tendency to give up too easily when something becomes too difficult. The concept of work is lost on young children, because without mixed feelings and thoughts, they are unable to delay gratification. In order to work, you need to forgo gratification and push through frustration that may arise.

A father of a four-year-old shared the following:

> I took my son golfing. He was having fun until he got frustrated when the ball didn't go where he wanted it. I told him to be patient, but he just got mad and threw down his club and said he quit. I told him to keep trying and to work at it, but he started to yell and scream. What am I supposed to do when he is like this? Is he lazy? He doesn't work at anything and just gives up when it's too hard. That's not what I want for him.

As the father realized his son was unable to persevere or work towards a goal, he softened in his expectations of him.

The best way to help young children persevere with a task is through play—the antithesis of work. Agendas that push work on them too early will backfire and can stir up frustration and resistance.

6. It's All about "Me" or "You" but Never "We"

Young children *only do one person at a time, and it is usually them*. Their attention will be on either themselves or another person, making them appear highly egocentric or an avid follower of other people. With room for only one person in mind, they cannot do togetherness without a loss of being a separate person. Young children don't move from "me" to "we"; they move from "me" to "you."

A young child begins to have a clear sense of self by age 2, but before this they do not see the world as being separate from themselves.[30] One of the goals of early childhood is to cultivate this emerging self and solidify it. Children will require space, time, and support to understand who they are instead of being preempted by the needs or desires of others. Preschooler integrity and selfhood are the prerequisites for participation as a community member in adulthood.

Young children will sometimes appear "inconsiderate" when they act in accordance with their own needs. They think nothing of telling someone, "Pick me up," despite that person's arms being full of groceries or other children. They can display deep concern for others too, giving away their possessions only to later demand, "I want them back!" The current emphasis in early childhood on getting along and considering the needs of others eclipses the more important developmental goal. Young children first need to understand who they are. Personal integration and the cultivation of selfhood come before social integration and interdependence.

Strategies for Dealing with the Immature

THE NATURE OF the young child is part Beauty and part Beast, leaving parents to long for the development of self-control, patience, and consideration. Although brain development cannot be hurried, there are a number of strategies for dealing with immaturity that will support growth and buy time until maturity provides the ultimate answer to impulsive, inconsiderate, and egocentric behaviour.

1. Supervision Is the Antidote to Immaturity

Adults can compensate for young children's immaturity by assuming responsibility for keeping them out of trouble through anticipating problems before they occur. Assuming a caretaking stance instead of a punitive one is key to managing immaturity. Young children don't do well on unsupervised playdates, sharing favourite toys, or figuring out park rules for themselves. They need adult supervision and direction when interacting with each other. The more parents make sense of young children, the more those parents will be able to predict when children are likely to get into trouble and get there first.

When trouble ensues, among the first questions to ask are whether the child was placed in a situation that was too much for them developmentally and whether expectations for behaviour were realistic. As parents reflect upon incidents, a child can reveal themselves in a new way, as one mother shared: "I took my child to an indoor play centre, but he started to melt down after an hour. In hindsight, I think it was actually too much for him. A half hour would have been better."

2. Use Structure and Routine to Orchestrate Behaviour

Structure and routine can compensate for a young child's lack of organizational and social abilities. When young children get used to a routine, less explicit directions are required and little room is left for improvisation. Structure and routine provide guidelines for behaviour and expectations, which help a young child appear more mature than they actually are. Given that young children lack perspective and operate with incomplete information, structure and routine will help compensate for their gaps in understanding. Routines can be part of everyday events, such as waking up, eating, and bedtime. Routines can help make things smoother, as the child knows what to predict at the same time each day, and routines also provide them with a sense of security. As one child care provider said, "We usually eat lunch in my kitchen, but for a change one day, I took the kids for a picnic in the backyard. When we came back inside, they all sat down at the kitchen table waiting to eat their lunch. It was like they couldn't move on with their day without going through all of our regular routine."

3. **Script the Actions of the Immature**

Young children can't read all the social cues or fully grasp what is expected of them in many situations. In scripting a young child, an adult purposively gives them cues, directions, or bearings in a situation where they might be confused or need to look "mature." For example, a parent can script a child's interactions for greeting someone: "A hug is a good idea, but not a kiss on the mouth." You can tell them ahead of time, "Preschool will involve sitting in a circle and putting up your hand to speak." If adults can anticipate and consider what new situations mean for a young child, they are better able to give them directions in advance for appropriate behaviour. If children are not attached to the adult giving the directions, they are unlikely to follow scripting instructions. Only strong relationships will activate a young child's desire to follow directions.

4. **Maintain an Alpha Position and Avoid Displacing Children's Emotions**

When a young child's emotions erupt or they behave immaturely, adults need to step in to manage the situation from their caretaking position. This is the case on the playground as much as it is in the home with sibling conflict. It is important in these situations to keep your relationship intact and not to displace one emotion in the young child for another. For example, when a young child is frustrated and lashes out, an adult may alarm them by yelling or threatening them to make them stop. The child's frustration may be replaced by fear, which can fan their emotional upset. Furthermore, when a parent displaces the child's original emotion, the moment is lost to help them understand what stirred the child up in the first place.

Most of children's problematic behaviour is driven by frustration or alarm, and to teach children words to replace hits, kicks, shoves, and yells, we need opportunities to connect impulses with "feeling" words. We can do this by acknowledging and reflecting children's feelings while giving words to their impulses. When we alarm a child in order to get compliance, we will probably thwart any understanding of what emotion they were experiencing before that. Displaced emotions can be unleashed on other children, pets, or toys. Chapter 6 addresses children's emotions, and chapter 7 focuses specifically on frustration and aggression.

5. **Support Conflict and Dissonance**

Adults can model for a young child how the brain will naturally integrate conflicting feelings and thoughts with phrases such as "Part of me feels this way, part of me wants to do something else," or "On the other hand…," or "I feel very mixed about this." When adults convey that it is okay to express internal conflict and dissonance, a child will start to get the message that there is merit in considering multiple perspectives and feelings in decision making.

The Onset of Mixed Thoughts and Feelings

PARENTS ROUTINELY ASK when they can expect to see signs of integration in feelings and thoughts, and what it looks like. Although the timing differs from child to child, there are a number of common signs that can start to appear as young as age 4 and increase in frequency as they near 5, with ideal development.

Reflection is one of the first signs that a young child's prefrontal cortex is transforming into a mixing bowl for conflicting thoughts or feelings. I asked a father if he saw any signs of contemplation in his four-and-a-half-year-old daughter, Maeve, and he said, "It's funny you ask this because I remember the other night when the waitress asked Maeve if she was done her dinner, Maeve looked up at her and paused and said, 'Maybe.' Maeve's eyes then looked sideways as if searching for an answer in her head. She then turned back to the waitress and said, 'Yes, my tummy says it is all done.' " Signs of reflection can appear subtly like this—a pause before proceeding, or a moment of silence before speaking. Spontaneous contemplation can start to occur around the age of 4, quickly appearing and disappearing. Adults can start to prime a child at this age by asking them what they think, but it shouldn't be forced, contrived, or made into a work project. Parents can just take comfort that there are signs of maturity appearing.

As the prefrontal cortex evolves into a mixing bowl, conflicting thoughts will appear before mixed feelings. Emotions are intense signals, making them more challenging to mix. As thoughts start to mix, a young child may make statements such as "Part of me wants to go to the park, but part of me wants to stay home." These contradictory statements indicate that the child can hold two conflicting thoughts at the same time. They may start to show amusement at hearing knock-knock jokes or puns, as one boy did: "Hey, Mommy, know what the cat says? It's purrrrrfect!"

A parent of a kindergartner told the following story, demonstrating the unfolding of mixed feelings:

> Mother: (Driving kids to school) "What are you going to tell the kids about your dream catcher for show and tell?"
>
> Tabitha: "I am not going to show them."
>
> Mother: "But at home you were so excited to tell the kids about your dream catcher. Are you scared? Is there one side of you excited to show it, but the other side is scared?"
>
> Tabitha: "Mama, no sides of me want to show those kids my dream catcher."

Although the mother was disappointed that fear and desire could not mix, she was delighted to hear that Tabitha had more than one side to her. Fear and desire are some of the hardest feelings to mix because of their intensity. When fear and desire can be felt at the same time, they will result in courage, which drives the capacity to move forward towards one's desire. Courage is not the absence of fear but, rather, fear balanced by desire.

As conflicting feelings and impulses start to mix, young children can spontaneously start to shake and shudder, grit their teeth, or show some other physical manifestations of conflict. One side may want to move away while the other side is moving towards; their inner tension is palpable. A mother of a five-and-a-half-year-old girl described this tension in her daughter: "The other day Amanda was frustrated and went to throw a train at her brother. I was shocked when she didn't throw it but held on to it as she started swinging her arms above her head, back and forth, to and fro. It was like one hand wanted to throw the train, but the other hand didn't. Sometimes she is able to stop herself, she is changing."

Conflicting feelings that start to mix may appear with expressions such as "I half hate you right now!" or "I half love you right now" or "I want to hit you but I won't." A mother of a four-and-a-half-year-old said,

Last week we were at a playground and Zach was surrounded by toddlers. One toddler gave Zach a shove. I started hurrying over, but Zach didn't move. He just looked at the toddler. That night, at bedtime, I started a conversation with him.

Mom: "I noticed a toddler pushed you today at the playground. You didn't push back. What was happening for you?"

Zach: "When he pushed me, all I felt was my caring."

Mom: "Your caring? Did you have any pushes in you?"

Zach: "No. No pushes. But I did have a hug in me for him."

Mom: "A hug?! Where did the hug come from?"

Zach: "Oh, Mama! That little guy was having a hard time. He needed a cuddle."

Mom: "Why didn't you give him that hug?"

Zach: "I thought that if I went to hug him, he'd push me again."

As the mother reflected on Zach's behaviour, she added, "I don't think I would have recognized how significant our conversation was without understanding mixed feelings. As well, I couldn't at first make sense of his 'paralysis'—why wasn't he moving? But I think he was stuck in 'hug him—don't hug him.' It's a baby step, but it feels incredibly important to me."

As young children's cognitive and emotional systems become increasingly integrated, their pendulum-like swings in behaviour will start to diminish. They will start to see two sides to the story and become more civilized as they interact with others. Although parents may rejoice at the tempering this brings, a young child will never be so pure or alone in their thoughts or feelings again. As a mother of a five-and-a-half-year-old girl stated,

> Anna was tormented by her mixed feelings and thoughts when they started to appear. She was trying to fall asleep one night and complained it wasn't fair her younger sister seemed to have an easier time than her. In anger, Anna looked at me and said, "I just can't sleep, my head just wants to think and think and think. How can I make it be quiet?" I managed to contain my excitement and told her that she was just getting a big-girl brain and it was just busier. Anna said in anger, "I don't want a big-girl brain. I just want to go to sleep like my sister."

In our eagerness to celebrate a young child's more civilized form, we can miss what will be lost. Gone will be the purity and innocence that comes with experiencing the world one thought or feeling at a time. No longer will their lives feel unfettered, unrestrained, and uncomplicated by choice. Why would a child be overjoyed to learn they will have a conscience that speaks to them regularly and that will give rise to conflicting thoughts and feelings? When the prefrontal cortex evolves into a mixing bowl, the organic solution to immaturity spontaneously appears, but that child's internal world will never be as peaceful or quiet again. However, there are important gains to be had from integration, as this father states: "I knew when my son no longer had a preschooler brain when he came to me with his hand in a fist and said proudly, 'Look, Daddy, look what I just did! I held my fist over Sara's head and wanted to thump her, but I didn't.' The look of pride on his face was amazing, like he was saying, 'I can't believe I can control this body of mine when I am frustrated.'" As the father relayed his story, it became clear how a child will experience such dignity in realizing their human potential as a tempered and self-controlled being.

Preserving Play
Defending Childhood in a Digital World

*It's our insides that make us who we are, that allow us to dream and
wonder and feel for others. That's what's essential. That's what will
always make the biggest difference in our world.*

FRED ROGERS[1]

A S A CHILD, Gail dreamed of having "magic scissors" that could
transform her drawings into real objects. Her father remarked
that her room "was always knee deep in paper clippings." A
lot of cutting ensued after Gail and her sister watched the film *Okla-
homa!* Gail's scissors brought to life cowboys, cowgirls, and a ranch
complete with horses and corrals; and with her sister, she disappeared into a fantasy world of their own making. The substance of
their adventures is hard to recollect, but for Gail the significance of
her play is clear. More than sixty years later, the creation of these
drawings tells part of the story of who Gail became and what she did
as her life's work.

Images played a special role in Gail's life and in her vocation
as an artist. They were vital to her well-being, and she expressed
herself intuitively through them. Gail was always a visual learner
and was bored by text and stories in school. She felt that images in
drawings or paintings were held captive and longed to be released

and understood. She saw her world as a matrix of images, and she separated each one out and brought it to life. Her drawing, cutting, sewing, pasting, sculpting, or forming imbued each image with deeper meaning.

As an adult, Gail followed her passion by studying ceramics in university. Gail dedicated most of her life to her art, working at the Emily Carr Institute of Art and Design (now Emily Carr University) until she retired. She was publicly honoured for her "lifelong contributions to the ceramics community and, particularly ceramics education."[2] Although Gail's "magic scissors" never materialized, they did help unfold a lifelong passion for images. It was this simple tool, along with enough space and freedom to play, that allowed Gail to discover the artist within her.

One is left to wonder who Gail would have become if she were raised today—at a time when instruction, structured activities, digital devices, and peer interaction are increasingly valued over the "empty hours" of endless play. As David Elkind, a psychologist and play advocate, states, "The decline of children's free, self-initiated play is the result of a perfect storm of technological innovation, rapid social change, and economic globalization."[3] The type of play young children require is being threatened with extinction in a digital world. This should be one of our greatest concerns, and should overshadow preoccupations with preschooler behaviour or discipline. Young children cannot thrive or flourish in a world without play; the very essence of who they will become is defined by it.

Play Is Endangered for Those Who Need It Most

PLAY SHOULD BE added to the endangered list, despite evidence from developmental science over the last 75 years demonstrating its critical importance for healthy growth in young children.[4] Developmental experts continue to sound alarm bells about the loss of play, but these voices struggle to outmatch parental, educational, governmental, and cultural pressures that push in the opposite direction.[5] Play is increasingly relegated to a young child's spare time rather than being the central focus of early childhood. Despite tacit agreement about the importance of play, many parents don't want to "risk" applying that lesson to their own kids for fear their children will get left behind.[6] But the growth that happens in play is not immediate or amenable to teaching or testing. The advances made are largely invisible, as selfhood and development unfold silently.

The type of play young children need is being eroded, crushed, and redefined by the onslaught of digital devices and early academics.[7] Daycare providers and preschool teachers face constant pressure from parents to teach their children to do math, read, and use technological devices. One early childhood educator said,

> I see families filling their child's days by doing many activities in the week, and their reasoning is that they are providing their child with skills to get ahead in the school years, getting a head start. I truly believe children who continue through their early years with busy lives do not understand pauses and feel the need to fill their spaces with white noise, thereby never really having an opportunity to rest.

The role of play in a young child's life is undervalued, underestimated, and unprotected when parents and educators push for outcomes. Play becomes suffocated under an adultcentric quest for speedier development, despite research demonstrating that children's brains reach the same cognitive benchmarks today as they did one hundred years ago.[8]

A further challenge is the influence on play of digital tools. With the increased availability of screens and educational programming, young children can entertain themselves like never before. A child's need to figure out something for themselves is supplanted by speedy access to information as well as by early academics that trump discovery. Children today are rescued from facing futility or loss in the videogame world where reset buttons, cheat codes, and endless lives are all possible. There is less room for boredom and the unexpected adventures that arise from it, something previous generations recall and, in hindsight, cherish.

There is no greater task in raising young children today than creating the conditions that will protect the space and time for play. It means pushing back against the cultural tide that sees play as frivolous and unproductive instead of as the bedrock upon which our children realize their full human potential. Without an understanding of how play serves development, it will be hard for adults to withstand the pressures to push ahead that undermine what children really need to grow.

What Is Play?

PLAY IS THE birthplace of personhood—it is how the self is born psychologically.[9] Play isn't about putting information into a child but about drawing out a child's ideas, intentions, aspirations, preferences, wants, and wishes. Play allows children to express themselves, despite their lack of words and understanding. It is in play that a young child hears the echo of what is within resonate in the world around them. Young children are natural learners driven to make sense of their environment and who they are in it. They need to emerge from early childhood with a sense of self that has been forged from hours spent lost in play. Play fosters development as a viable, separate being as it unearths a child's interests, desires, and goals. It moves a child from depending upon adults and unlocks the desire to venture forth, discover, or make sense of their experiences. Play is where the spirit that underlies growth is revealed and vitality is expressed. In short, play is the act of self-creation.

The type of play young children need is characterized by freedom, enjoyment, and a leap into settings to explore. They need bounded spaces in which to freely move, with perimeters formed by the adults who care for them. Play is a spontaneous act that arises from a particular state of mind—you can't teach or command a child to play. There are three essential characteristics to play: it is (1) not work, (2) not for real, and (3) expressive and exploratory. This definition can be used to evaluate what activities truly foster ideal conditions for play.

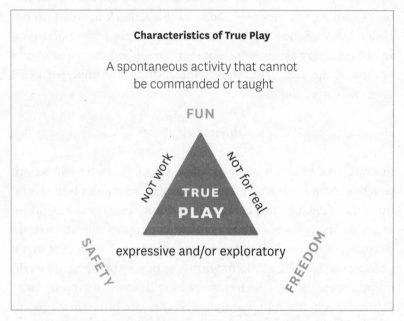

Figure 3.1 Adapted from Neufeld *Making Sense of Play* course

1. Play Is Not Work

Young children are built for play and ill suited for work. Goals, *performance, worksheets,* and *expectations* are the language of work, whereas *freedom, imagination, fun,* and *discovery* are associated with play. When a child is playing, their focus should be on the activity rather than on any particular outcome as set by an adult or another child. Adults can take any activity and turn it into work by changing what engages a child's attention. For example, playing a musical instrument for fun is different from having to practise for a recital. If a child draws and an adult suggests that the art needs to look a certain way or that it will be used as a gift, they will shift the child's attention towards outcome. This also happens frequently at dinner tables when a parent focuses on getting food into their young child rather than on preserving mealtimes as fun and appealing.

Play is where the fun happens. By contrast, when one is working on something, the "fruits of one's labour" are enjoyed upon *completing* a task. For example, my niece and nephew used to love to play with duct tape. Their mother gave them scissors as well as an array of colours and patterns to choose from. She also gave them a few rules, to create a bounded space, rules such as no taping each other, any pets, or items in the house. They played happily for hours, creating purses, wallets, and bookmarks. They even created a storefront named Duct Tape Delights. As friends and family visited their house, the orders for camouflage wallets, bacon- and pickle-patterned purses, and polka-dot bookmarks increased. Their "customers" told them they should sell their creations and make real money. But as Taylor and Jamie felt the pressure to fill orders and focus on outcomes, the delight and fun diminished.

When children are at play, they are focused, engaged, and having fun in experiencing the activity. When we push for outcomes, or have predetermined goals and expectations, we turn their play into work. As Mark Twain said, "Work consists of whatever a body is obliged to do. Play consists of whatever a body is not obliged to do."[10]

2. Play Is Not for Real

Play is meant to happen outside the realities of everyday life. It is supposed to be consequence- and risk-free so that a child can play without being focused on any particular result. While at play, children use their internal world to create a new setting, through imagination and fantasy. As one mother wrote, "I watch my daughter become a chef, designer, teacher, and dancer, shape shifting before my eyes." Play is where the dress rehearsal for life happens—it should never be judged as being either right or wrong. It is where a child can get married and separated as many times as they like without facing financial ruin and heartache. It is where they can vent their emotions yet experience few repercussions. For example, a mother said, "My kids were screaming and yelling at each other, so I yelled for them to stop and tell me what was going on. They looked at me with surprise and said, 'But Mom, we're only play fighting.' " When a child is playing, it shouldn't count for anything other than what it means to them.

3. Play Is Expressive and Exploratory

Play is not a passive experience in which a child is made to be a bystander. In play, a child places a hand on the steering wheel of their own life and becomes an active agent in discovering and exploring. Children at play should express themselves using objects, people, or spaces, rather than being led by someone else's colouring lines or algorithms. Play involves the outflow of energy from the child—the antithesis of boredom, where nothing moves from within. A child should naturally play with numbers, lines, sounds, words, or ideas. When children receive instruction, attend structured activities, or engage with digital devices, there is little freedom to draw out their expression and explore freely. As one mother explained,

> I love watching my children when they are deep in play, dressed up in incredibly creative and expressive outfits. The best seems to be when they use simple things: scarves, bits of cloth, and accessories. My son was recently playing being a pirate on our deck/ship. He was alone, full of all kinds of sounds and actions of a "real" pirate battle. The noise of his stomping and heave-ho-ing and battle cries was so "real," I could almost feel the ship/deck rocking in the sea!

Children need to discover their own story in play rather than being overwhelmed with the stories of so many others.

We often say our children are playing even when there are outside goals imposed on this time and consequences when it comes to performance, both of which serve to diminish exploration and expression. To create real opportunities for children to play, we need to make sure their engagement in an activity doesn't include a focus on outcomes, isn't inhibited by the fear of real-life consequences, and doesn't make them passive recipients of information or instruction.

What Is the Purpose of Play?

G. STANLEY HALL, an early writer on adolescence, wrote, "Men grow old because they stop playing, and not conversely."[11] Play is essential to healthy human functioning over the lifespan but critical for development in the early years because it is (1) where the self is truly expressed, (2) where growth and development take place, and (3) where psychological health and well-being are preserved.

1. Play Is Where the Self Is Truly Expressed

At age 4, Nolan told his mother he wanted to be a taxi driver when he grew up. He loved to sing and drive his toy cars up and down the stairs, in and out of the bathtub, or into the garden. Nolan's mother was aghast and told him, "You don't want to be a taxi driver. This

WHY CHILDREN NEED TO PLAY

- to forward development and realize their potential
- to find and express their true selves
- to program the brain's problem solving networks
- to preserve psychological health and well-being
- to find their creative edge and responsibility
- to practise life in a space free of consequences

Figure 3.2 Adapted from Neufeld *Making Sense of Play* course

isn't a good job and you won't make very much money." Nolan continued to drive his cars and told his mother weeks later, "I want to be a singer." Again, his mother was aghast and told him this was another bad career decision and he needed to go to university. What his mother missed was how Nolan's self was emerging through envisioning his future. He had begun to experiment, grasping the steering wheel in his own life and pointing in a direction of his own choosing. The response he got was his vision was disappointing and unacceptable. What Nolan needed was a shame-free environment in which to learn, express, and create. He needed the spirit that was driving him to become his own person to be celebrated regardless of its form. At age 4, he needed his adults to understand that his experimentation with form wasn't as important as whether there was a self emerging in the first place.

Nolan's story underlines a recurring and heartbreaking theme when it comes to young children today. We have become preoccupied with the form children take—as learners, as friends, in their behaviour or conduct, and in how they meet adult expectations. The developmental feat personhood represents is lost, replaced with fixations on whether children are measuring up and achieving. Play is where children express their true selves and come forward as separate beings. This is why the emphasis in play needs to be on their desires, want-to's, curiosity, intentions, initiatives, aspirations, expression, and personal meanings. If adults make demands on their playtime, deliver instruction, or focus on behaviour, they *crush* the emerging self. If we are to preserve the spirit of childhood through play, we cannot make our children perform for us based on our own needs and desires.

The drive to become one's own person is captured well in three-year-old Aiden's statement to his mother. She interrupted him while playing by saying, "Come on, honey, we need to go to the store." Aiden turned around with his hands on his hips and proudly declared, "Don't call me 'honey,' I am not your honey—I am Aiden!"

I often think that if we are going to preserve the spirit of childhood, we need to give every two- or three-year-old who says "Me-do" or "I do it myself" a special celebration to reflect their psychological arrival into personhood. It would help us pause long enough to realize that the words "I am" are nothing short of a developmental miracle.

2. Play Is Where Brain Growth and Development Take Place

Jean Piaget, the Swiss developmental psychologist, once asked, "Are we forming children who are only capable of learning what is already known? Or should we try to develop creative and innovative minds, capable of discovery from the preschool age on, throughout life?"[12] If lifelong learning, creativity, and innovation are desired in a knowledge-based global economy, then play is surely the answer. Healthy young children are creative, are full of questions, and problem solve while playing. As one grandmother said, "My grandson is two and he is always asking me, 'Why?' If I answer him he just asks another 'why' question."

When children are playing, their brains are being sculpted by their interactions with the environment.[13] Stuart Brown, a psychiatrist and founder of the National Institute for Play, states that the complexity of the brain is enhanced most of all by hours spent in play—play is nature's answer to growth. As neurons fire together, they form stronger pathways, because the brain operates on a use-it-or-lose-it system.[14] Motor, perceptual, cognitive, social, and emotional areas of the brain integrate or wire up when a child plays. Complex networking systems are built and become the basis for problem solving used in school and adulthood.[15]

When young children play, they engage in trial and error and form new relationships between objects.[16] Critical thinking, communication, language, self-expression, and cognitive skills are all developed through play. As children touch and explore objects by hand, they are able to ground abstract ideas in the concrete world.[17]

Impairments to cognitive, language, emotional, and physical development have all been linked to a deficit in play.[18]

Play is where creativity is also most likely to be expressed. For example, a father said, "My son wanted to play with his big cars and little trains at the same time but was troubled by the size difference. He finally said the cars were created by the giants and the little people rode in the trains." Another parent said, "I walked into my daughter's room to find she had taken the blue sticky tack out of my drawer and had stuck candy to the wall. She told me it was her candy wall so it was close whenever I said she could have one." Another child told her father, "I chomped my pretzel into a D for Daddy and left it under your pillow." A five-year-old planning his hamster's birthday party said, "I want the party to have a cage-like feeling so we need to have it under the table and put blankets over it to cover it."

Children are some of the most creative and curious people in the world. When children have their own ideas and questions, we will be able to teach them many things. We cannot, however, teach a child to be creative and curious. This is cultivated in play, where a sense of agency and responsibility is forged in a consequence-free environment.

3. Play Preserves Psychological Health and Well-Being

Play is therapeutic for young children because it allows them to express deep emotions safely. In pretend places and fantasy worlds, there should be little repercussion for expressing frustration, fear, sadness, disappointment, or jealousy. In play, a young child's brain works to release and make sense of emotional content. It serves to balance their emotional system, which is routinely stirred up throughout the day.

Play also serves emotional development by helping a child understand their inner world by making it visible. According to Joe Frost, a professor and play advocate for more than 50 years, play allows a child to turn what is not understood into something manageable. As children play out their emotions, the images and impulses emerge at a distance, despite a lack of words or conscious awareness.[19]

Neuroscientist Jaak Panksepp states that we ought to foster play sanctuaries for young children as a means of promoting emotional and mental health.[20] He says young children's urge to play is built into the emotional centres of the brain and could be the most underused resource for dealing with their feelings. In fact, play preserves emotional functioning in all mammal species and helps reduce stress and boredom as well as cultivate resiliency.[21] Child development experts have linked a lack of play with anxiety, attention problems, and depression in young children,[22] and a lack of play in preschool years has been linked with emotional and social problems in adulthood.[23]

Parents often remark on the stories that emerge in their child's play, from mundane experiences to revelations of internal conflict. One mother said, "It was a bit of a joke between my husband and me that we could predict what form the play was going to take based on what we had been doing as a family. After we got back from the zoo, our basement became a zoo. After we got back from the store, our basement became the store." Another parent said that when his daughter started kindergarten, she played teacher, lining up her dolls, with some being scolded while others listened patiently as she made up stories for them.

When a child is stirred up, their play can reflect the themes they are struggling with. Parents of alpha children (see chapter 5) often notice that play contains undercurrents of dominance and dependency, as evident in one five-year-old. A parent was confused by her son's obsessive play in which he repeatedly excluded himself from the rest of the family. She said, "Max creates an island in the middle of the living room and sets up a tent-like structure. He takes everything he needs to live there by himself, like food from the kitchen, his pillow and blankets, his toys and books. He won't let anyone come onto his island. It's like he hides or runs away there." When the parent understood that Max's isolation was a move made out of desperation, she was able to start answering his underlying emotional needs. Although play can appear lighthearted, its underlying emotional themes are serious business.

In play, pictures are drawn, structures are made, and games are engaged in to allow emotions to come out from underneath defences without evoking too much vulnerability. Five-year-old Clayton was struggling with separation from his mother because of her cancer treatment. His father noticed that Clayton always wanted to play a dog-fighting game with him. He began to play with him every night and was surprised it seemed to help with his frustration, anxiety, and sleep issues.

> Every night we play this game where I am the big daddy dog and he is the grumpy puppy. He growls and charges at me for close to 45 minutes. He snips, snarls, and tries to bite me but doesn't hurt. I pin him down and he wrestles to get free. We do this over and over until he is exhausted. I know when he is done because he will curl up in my lap and whimper like a wounded puppy. I just hold him until he is done, telling him Daddy dog will take care of him.

The father seemed embarrassed that this simple game was his solution to his son's turmoil, but he had intuitively discovered how play is a perfect safety valve for a child's troubled emotional world.

Fostering the Freedoms Necessary for Play

PLAY IS ONE thing young children should know how to do really well, but they must have the necessary freedoms to ensure that play can occur. Current estimates of play time demonstrate it is on the decline, suffocated by a host of competing activities in addition to schooling. Sociologists Sandra Hofferth and John Sandberg found that between 1981 and 1997 there was a 25 percent reduction in time children spent playing.[24] They also measured a 55 percent reduction in time engaged in conversation at home, a 19 percent reduction in television watching, an 18 percent increase in time spent at school, a 145 percent increase in time spent on schoolwork at home, and a 168 percent increase in time spent with parents shopping. Play is competing against increasing academics, structured activities, and consumer-focused activities.

For children to truly play, they must have certain freedoms. This includes having their basic needs met, so that they have, for example, freedom from pain, hunger, or being tired. They also need freedom from instruction and schooling. Many parents don't want to push their child academically but worry about how that child will measure up to other kids if they do not. A mother said to me, "When my daughter was in kindergarten, I realized she was one of the last kids to read. I started to worry because I hadn't pushed her to read but to love books instead. I worried she was going to get left behind, but I just couldn't bring myself to make her read. I am so glad I didn't because by grade 4 she told me she was one of the few kids that still liked to read in her class." Not only parents feel the pressure to push academics in the early years; early childhood educators do as well, as one teacher told me:

> Children need time to just be kids, but there is an overemphasis in many preschools and kindergarten classes on getting students reading or learning math as soon as possible. The principal at my school expects students to be learning academics in kindergarten, despite that being there all day is already hard enough for them. It is also stressful because the parents expect this too.

Developmental readiness for schoolwork must be taken into consideration before a child is exposed to instruction and academics.

Young children need freedom from structured activities in which external forces dictate their actions and impinge upon their expression. Pediatrician Kenneth Ginsburg argues that enrichment activities are investments that do little to nourish the child–adult relationship.[25] Overscheduling leads to stress, anxiety, and a decrease in creativity. A hurried lifestyle does not favour conditions that give rise to play, requiring parents to take into account matters of balance where structured activities are concerned.

According to a report produced by the Campaign for a Commercial Free Childhood and the Alliance for Childhood, children are now introduced to screens in infancy.[26] Close to 30 percent of children under the age of 1 are watching television or videos for approximately 90 minutes a day. More than 60 percent of children between the ages of 1 and 2 are watching television or videos for more than 2 hours a day. Conservative estimates of screen time for young children aged 2 to 5 are more than 2 hours per day, whereas some research puts it as high as 4.5 hours per day. This persists despite guidelines from the American Academy of Pediatrics discouraging screen time for children under the age of 2 and limiting it for those older than 2.[27] Concern over the effects of screen time on early brain growth and the development of social, emotional, and cognitive skills is behind recommendations to limit or reduce that time.

The additional screen time young children are exposed to is interfering with basic needs, such as sleep, and is linked to obesity and with attention, learning, and social problems. Time spent watching television has not decreased among young children despite the

THE FREEDOM TO PLAY

- · enough freedom from pain and hunger and tiredness
- · enough freedom from instruction and schooling
- · enough freedom from scheduled activities
- · enough freedom from screens and entertainment
- · enough freedom from peers and siblings
- · enough freedom from having to work at attachment

Figure 3.3 Adapted from Neufeld *Making Sense of Play* course

increased use of other screens and devices.[28] Furthermore, when a child is in front of a screen, they are not engaging with parents or other people. The nature deficit argued by Richard Louv in his book *Last Child in the Woods* links a lack of outdoor play in particular with an increased use of digital devices.[29] In a six-year period from 1997 to 2003, the amount of time a child spent playing outside decreased by 50 percent.[30] A recovery effort is underway encouraging North American parents to get children to play outside and experience nature.[31]

Research on parents who grew up exposed to digital devices shows that they are more likely to let their young children play with their mobile device so that they can get chores done and run errands, to keep them calm in public, and to put them to sleep.[32] An early childhood educator said, "In the preschool group I lead, I see children getting frustrated, as they often do at this age. Parents are quick to take out their smartphone and give it to their child. I wonder how much additional screen time this means and what happens when a parent can't deal with their child's upset any other way?" The emergence of electronic devices to entertain children renders children passive recipients, as they typically lack the opportunity for open-ended exploration.[33] In short, screen time should be put into developmental perspective: young children need real-life experiences with real people, making parents the best devices out there.

The type of play young children need is often that which is done on their own without parents or peers as playmates. When children play together, it is usually left to one child to lead the play, while the others become passive recipients of direction and ideas. A young child needs to have time to become immersed in their own world for the purpose of expression or exploration. Parents often think they need to play with their child, and although this is not harmful, it is typically serving their child's relational needs. It is important to bear in mind that young children under the age of 3 have a minimal capacity to play on their own because of intense relational needs.

Like an elastic band that can stretch only so far, they need to return to their home attachment base to fill up on contact and closeness before venturing forth to play again. As a child becomes more deeply attached and develops as a separate person, they should be able to play on their own for longer stretches of time.

The biggest source of freedom a young child needs is the gift of deep relationships with parents or caretakers. In the hierarchy of a child's needs, attachment is the greatest and most necessary source of freedom for true play to unfold. A child needs to be at rest in their relationships so that their hunger for contact and closeness is satiated. They need enough love to feel content and enough significance to feel important. Cultivating the type of relationships that lead to rest is explored more deeply in chapters 4 and 5 but is addressed throughout *Rest, Play, Grow*.

Strategies for Promoting
the Conditions That Give Rise to Play

IF "SPONTANEOUS PLAY is the delicate dance of childhood that strengthens the mind and body,"[34] then how do we encourage a child to spend their time playing? The following are four key strategies that help set the stage for true play to unfold.

1. Answer Their Hunger for Contact and Closeness

Playtime needs to be prefaced with contact and closeness from an attachment figure so that a young child's relational needs are satiated. It is helpful to think of a young child as having an attachment fuel tank that needs to be topped up to overflowing before play can happen. Their attachment tanks can quickly get depleted, especially from ages 2 to 3 and for more sensitive kids. As a parent provides for their attachment needs, they can wait until the child pushes them away, suggesting they are full. One mother explained it this way:

After a few days of trying things, I learned how to help Oliver, my two-and-a-half-year-old, experience true play. When he was rested, fed, and had lots of attention from me, I cuddled him until he seemed to want to push away. I then asked him if he wanted to play and put him down on the floor. I found I had to stay in the same room with him, as he checked on me a couple of times, and I couldn't be doing anything interesting or directly watching him, as that would have distracted his attention. When he had enough, he would crawl back to me for more attention and cuddling. I would read a book or we would do something else together, and then he would push me away again. I was astonished how well he could play by himself when I simply gave him what he needed and waited until he backed away.

2. Create Voids to Be Filled Up

One of the prerequisites for play to unfold is space and time where competing activities are nonexistent and peer or sibling contact is limited. Play that is exploratory and expressive is often done by a child on their own when their agendas can take the lead and be at the fore. Children need to have access to materials for play, and room to explore and express themselves. This could be as simple as having paper, blocks, cars, or a backyard with sticks and mud. An adult will need to make room for a child's initiative, creativity, and originality, putting them in charge of their play whenever possible. One father said, "I was reading the paper while my kids played in the garden. My wife had given them a patch of dirt and said they could do whatever they wanted with it. They seemed happy enough, so I just read. When I looked up again, I saw they had picked a lot of my wife's flowers from the rest of the garden and stuck them in their patch of dirt." The father said he contemplated for some time how he was going to explain to his wife that benign neglect was really good for his children's development.

Furthermore, a child's interests should be given the lead in play as opposed to an adult's agenda. One mother said,

> My husband is an avid mountain bike rider and was eager to teach my daughter how to ride. When she got her new bike, he tried to get her to ride it, but she just wanted to play with the streamers and wash it. She eventually told her dad she wanted to walk it around the block, and as they did, she stopped every ten steps to take a sip out of her water bottle and put it carefully back in the cup holder. She thoroughly enjoying playing with her new bike, but my husband was utterly dismayed because she didn't want to ride it.

As the father was helped to see that his daughter's agenda for play was more important than his agenda, he was able to let go of his expectations and take delight in his daughter's enjoyment.

3. Create Structure, Ritual, and Routine to Protect Play

Play is not urgent, and therefore is easily lost in the activities of daily life. To protect and preserve time and space for play, use routines or rituals. For example, a parent can decide how many playdates, if any, should take place in a given week. A parent can create a daily routine that will balance out structured activities with playtime, making sure play doesn't get pushed to the side. When it comes to the use of digital devices, simple rituals governing when, where, how, and why they are used can help limit exposure and preempt problems. Devices are best left out of young children's bedrooms and should not be used as a reward or withheld as punishment. If they are out of sight, they will be out of mind for young children.

4. Don't Preempt Play with Praise or Rewards

The more an adult tries to reinforce play through praise and rewards, the more they may prevent it from unfolding. When a parent tells a child that they are proud of their play or the outcome of it, they can turn their play into a pursuit for attachment. This can be easily remedied by acknowledging how proud a child feels of their own accomplishment or how pleased a child is to have done something for themselves. The keys are not to use praise to manipulate behaviour and to be aware that true play needs space to unfold. When a child is truly lost in play, benign neglect can be the best approach, as one parent exemplified in the following story:

> My son used to sit at the piano with his sister and ask her what song she would like him to play. One day he gave her two choices— "Puff the Magic Dragon" or the song about a land named Agatera. Skylar told him she wanted the Agatera song. My son obliged, and even though he doesn't take piano lessons, he made up a song about a land named Agatera to the tune of "Puff the Magic Dragon." I was on the verge of laughing, as well as praising him for being so creative. I didn't end up saying anything because I was afraid of interrupting their play.

Play can be promoted only when adults value it and see it is a basic need for children. Play is not urgent, and its importance has become camouflaged by preoccupations with performance, immediate outcomes, and getting ahead. Adults need to buffer against technological innovation, rapid social change, and economic globalization—and against their own anxiety about their children's success that threatens to suffocate play. Children must lose themselves in play in order to discover who they are.

What Are the Implications for Work and Education in the Early Years?

GIVEN THE NEED for play in the early years, the question is often asked, when is a young child ready to work and start formal education? The answer is, when their brain is sufficiently developed—typically between the ages of 5 and 7, with ideal development. When a child is capable of mixed feelings and thoughts, they will have the impulse control they need to successfully participate in settings requiring patience, consideration, and focused attention (see chapter 2). The capacity for work requires a child to delay gratification, be capable of sacrifice, and forgo enjoyment to focus on an outcome. For example, a six-year-old told his mother he didn't like grade 1 "because they have desks and I have to sit and do work. I want to play and jump around, but I have to sit or my teacher will get mad at me." Clearly, he was ready to be in school because he could feel and express his mixed feelings.

Research has examined the efficacy of starting formal schooling at age 7. Delaying kindergarten to age 7 in the United States and Denmark was found to dramatically reduce the number of students who were likely to demonstrate attention and hyperactivity problems, thus increasing student achievement.[35] The delay in formal schooling allowed a young child's brain to integrate in the prefrontal areas, giving rise to focused attention and impulse control. In other words, maturity, not early academic instruction, is the answer to student success.

Until a child enters the "age of reason," we would do well to interject fun into any activity that could be construed as work, such as picking up toys, cleaning up, toilet training, hygiene tasks, or learning about numbers and letters. For example, one mother said, "I used food colouring to make toilet training more playful. I would get my son to choose the colour, then put a few drops in the bowl, and he would pee over it and make the water turn a different colour. It was a lot of fun, and it completely solved any resistance he had to toilet training."

One of the biggest issues in education today is the preservation of play in preschool and kindergarten settings. Play-based education, rather than instruction or academics, should be the focus at this age; however, this focus is increasingly under threat. The need to defend the early years from academics and instruction has become a global issue, from the United States to New Zealand. Early instruction and schooling is being rapidly introduced in some countries, with three- and four-year-olds learning math and English through formal instruction. Peter Gray, a psychologist and author of *Free to Learn*, states that preschools and kindergartens have become the final battlegrounds for the preservation of early childhood.[36]

The National Association for the Education of Young Children states that U.S. Common Core standards have pushed early academics in a belief that they foster job and college readiness.[37] In the United Kingdom, the Professional Association for Childcare and Early Years argues that early academics should not be the focus of preschool; instead, early childhood should be a time to foster creativity, encourage a desire for learning, and help a child become increasingly independent.[38] In New Zealand, the early childhood curriculum referred to as Te Whariki was created out of the Maori people's focus on childhood as a time *of* life instead of preparation *for* life.[39] Even countries such as Iceland and Sweden, known for their core values of play in the early years, are facing pressure to introduce academic subjects into preschool.[40] Fortunately, countries such as Denmark and Finland, as well as Canada, remain strong supporters of play as the best environment for children under the age of 6 or 7. Finland has received much attention for performing among the top countries in the OECD's Programme for International Student Assessment (PISA) measurement of education systems worldwide.[41] Finnish children are provided with a strong play-based education, and academics are typically introduced after the age of 6.[42]

Canada also ranked high in the PISA measurement of worldwide education systems before all-day kindergarten was implemented, while play-based education was the norm.[43] The shift to all-day kindergarten has been touted as a means of giving young children an academic advantage but has failed to produce results to this effect. In evaluations of the implementation of the Full-Day Early Learning–Kindergarten Program in Ontario, academic improvements have been minor, inconsequential, and even in favour of half-day kindergarten.[44] These findings support what Duke University researchers found in their meta-analysis of all-day kindergarten programs: no long-term academic benefits of all-day kindergarten programs as measured in grade 3. They concluded that all-day kindergarten should be available for children to attend but not universally required.[45] Research does support that early education and all-day kindergarten best serve the needs of children whose parents are unable to provide the conditions for true play.[46]

Research on the efficacy of early academics for young children has consistently come up short. Despite early literacy programs for preschoolers in the UK, children's reading skills are some of the lowest in Europe, lower than countries where children start reading at later ages.[47] There is no evidence globally to suggest reading at age 5 leads to greater academic success.[48] Furthermore, pushing academics too soon can negatively impact a child's disposition and motivation to learn.[49] Making a child read at age 5 can create stress and can be experienced as coercive. Children's natural desire to make sense of their world becomes stifled by worksheets, assessments, and classrooms, allowing for little exploration and expression. The early push for academics has been linked to a decrease in curiosity and creativity—casualties in the rush for knowledge and learning.[50] Young children who attended academic preschools displayed more test anxiety, showed less creativity, and viewed school more negatively than did kids who attended play-based preschools.[51]

There is a steady and alarming trend to push young children into academics, ignoring assertions from developmental science that instruction at this age is too early, too much, and undermines healthy growth. We can help young children reach their full human potential as students, but it will be through play and not at the expense of it. As child development expert Nancy Carlsson-Paige states, "Never in my wildest dreams could I have imagined that we would have to defend children's right to play."[52]

4

Hungry for Connection
Why Relationships Matter

There is no safe investment. To love at all is to be vulnerable.
Love anything, and your heart will certainly be wrung and possibly be
broken. If you want to make sure of keeping it intact, you must give your
heart to no one, not even to an animal. Wrap it carefully round
with hobbies and little luxuries; avoid all entanglements; lock it up safe
in the casket or coffin of your selfishness. But in that casket—safe,
dark, motionless, airless—it will change. It will not be broken; it will
become unbreakable, impenetrable, irredeemable.

C.S. LEWIS[1]

PENELOPE WAS A three-year-old I encountered while playing with my children at the park one day. After we had played marbles together, it was clear she intended to follow us wherever we went. When I asked her who was taking care of her, she pointed across the park to a woman who was engaged in conversation with another adult. A little bit later, I told Penelope she needed to return to her adult. She looked at me defiantly, but after some insistence on my part, I shuffled her off in her caretaker's direction. I returned my focus to my own children, only to suddenly feel a little hand grasp mine. Shocked, I looked down to see her standing there again. She told me she wanted to come with me. I told her again she needed to find her adult and waved to get her caretaker's attention. Ten minutes later, Penelope found me again, but this time she was crying, "Swing, swing, swing." I took Penelope and approached her caretaker, interrupted her conversation, and told her Penelope was upset because she wanted to go on the swing. Her caretaker looked at me flatly and said, "Yes, she is upset because she wants you to push her on the swing." Stunned, angry, and confused, I couldn't believe her caretaker's response. I was a stranger to this child, and there was nothing healthy about her pursuit of me. I told Penelope her caretaker would push her on the swings and I had to go watch *my* children. I walked away upset as I listened to Penelope cry, angered that her caretaker lacked any desire to assume responsibility for her.

Penelope's behaviour was fuelled by a hunger for contact and closeness. She was starving relationally and willing to pursue any stranger who offered her the possibility of warmth and connection. Although part of me yearned to take care of her, I knew I could not aid her in her pursuit of strangers, as it wouldn't serve her overall. Penelope was not at fault; she was only being true to her instincts to find a person with whom she felt at "home." The irony was that Penelope was not without the comforts of home. She was well dressed; she had a nice wagon, a beautiful park, and a safe neighbourhood to play in. Most people would look at her and believe that she was doing well and getting what she needed to grow. The reality was that Penelope wasn't doing well and was famished.

Penelope's story demonstrates the challenge of attachment: its otherwise invisible nature is revealed only when one has eyes to see it or is moved by caring instincts to respond to it. Her story also highlights how children will work at getting their attachment needs met when a provider doesn't assume responsibility for this. Children are not meant to work for love. They are meant to rest in someone's care so that they can play and grow; this is why relationships matter.

The Hunger for Connection and the Invitation for Rest

T.S. ELIOT WROTE, "Home is where one starts from,"[2] but what makes a young child feel at home in the first place? Children don't simply feel at home wherever they are planted—they must be rooted through attachment. A sense of home is more than just a geographical location or physical structure; it is an emotional place where a child finds rest from the hunger for connection. Children need relational homes, but we cannot command this; we need to invite them into relationship and invite them to rest in our care. We cannot give explicit directions on how to love or care for another person; rather, we can support the idea that being attached is the answer to our greatest hunger as human beings.

More than 60 years of attachment research has demonstrated that what every child needs is at least one strong, caring adult to attach to. Attachment is defined as *the drive or relationship characterized by the pursuit and preservation of proximity.*[3] We seek to keep close the things or people we are attached to. For healthy development to unfold, young children need to attach to their caretakers, but they can also attach to objects and other people, from teddy bears to grandparents. There is no such thing as being too attached, just not being attached deeply enough. The attachment instinct is fuelled by the limbic system, also referred to as the emotional centre of the brain.[4] Attachment's chemical traces include oxytocin and vasopressin, which are believed to have a superglue-like force, binding us to each other.[5]

Attachment is the preeminent need of a young child. Their innate *seeking instinct* moves them to search for people who are the answer to the question: Who will take care of me?[6] The seeking instinct propels a child forward in forming strong attachments that will feed their relational hunger and provide a *secure base* in which to feel at home.[7] It is not *a parent's* love for a child that empowers them in their caretaking role, but *the child's* attachment to their parent. Five-year-old Simone described this well over a picnic lunch with her mother:

Simone: "I am so glad to be alive, Mama."
Mother: "Me too. Why do you feel that way?"
Simone: "Because I have you."
Mother: "I know exactly what you mean."

A parent needs to work at attachment so that a child can take their invitation to rest for granted.

Whenever a child is hurt or scared, it is their relational home they should seek, as the mother of four-year-old Chloe explained: "Whenever Chloe is really upset she cries out, 'I want to go home ... I want to go home ...' I was really confused at first and would point out to her that she was in her house, but she just cried even louder and said, 'I want to go home to Mama.' She seems lost at these times and just wants the comfort of my arms."

It is also no accident young children have built in "homing devices" that set off alarm signals whenever they are apart from their caretakers and in need of attention. A mother of two young boys said, "Whenever I get on the phone, my boys start to circle me like sharks. They tug, they pull, they fight and scream until I get off and pay attention to them. I can't get a minute to myself." Young children are creatures of attachment, and missing this fact would eclipse understanding what fuels much of their behaviour.

The young child's all-consuming, seeking, hungry pursuit of their caretaker is nothing new. In 1958, John Bowlby, the British psychiatrist who coined this use of the word *attachment*, told parents, "The young child's hunger for his mother's love and presence is as great as his hunger for food."[8] He said to expect young children to make relentless demands of parents, especially when they're frightened or upset. Bowlby argued that this was a natural process, and that although parents may feel overwhelmed and tired at times, the demands of the child should decrease with healthy development and a more secure child should emerge. When you realize how big the attachment needs of a young child are, you realize how much generosity is required of a parent.

Dorothy Briggs wrote in her book *Your Child's Self-Esteem*, "You nourish from overflow; not emptiness."⁹ It is the overflow that matters most when it comes to satiating the hunger for attachment. It is with a generous provision of care that we invite our children into relationship and provide for them. It is because of abundance that a child is free to rest in our care and take us for granted. Our generosity is the perfect match to their hunger for contact and closeness, pulling them into orbit around us. A five-year-old named Sofia conveyed to her mother how she experienced the generosity of her caretaking and its impact on her:

> Sometimes I have this dream when I am waking up that I have a love scale and so do you. Your love scale is always higher than mine, so I try really hard to push it up higher to reach yours. Just when I get there, yours always jumps up more. I try to push my love scale higher and higher to reach yours, but every time I do, yours always gets bigger again. I just can't keep up to your love, Mama.

As the mother listened, she realized that her invitation to relationship had trumped her daughter's pursuit of connection.

The shape and expression of a generous invitation to attachment will change according to each situation. For example, if a young child asks for a hug, a parent may give them five, but when they are upset by a parent's no's, generosity may mean making room for the tears they need to shed. Whatever the scenario, we need to invite our children into relationship by pursuing and holding on to them—through both the storms and the good times. Satisfying the intense attachment hunger of a young child is a tall order for any parent, but feed them we must.

The early years are hungry ones. Young children are restless seekers who are satiated only when allowed to feast on human connection. Attachment is a primal quest, and a strong, caring, generous adult is the ultimate answer to its achievement. Although most parents, teachers, grandparents, and care providers intuitively agree on the importance of adult–child relationships, I am routinely asked the following:

· How do you build strong attachments with children?

· Can you be too attached?

· If you had problems with attachment as a child, can you still attach to your child?

· Is it bad if I didn't attach to my child right away when they were born?

· Can I work and leave my kids in daycare and still have a strong relationship with them?

· What if I am a single parent and all they have is me?

· How do I get them to attach to their teacher? grandparents? siblings?

These questions are heartening, as they signal a shift in focus towards relationships between children and adults. What needs further clarification is who is meant to feed children relationally, how they need to be fed, and how this serves their development. What is clear is that adults are responsible for meeting a child's relational hunger. It is a parent's response to their child's need for contact and closeness that influences the trajectory of growth and the realization of human potential.

What Does a Good Attachment Look Like?

ONE OF THE things my grandfather was proudest of when it came to his garden was his soil. He treasured his dark, rich earth, a concoction of composted material he constantly experimented with that contained "the secret to growth." As a child I cared very little about his dirt and paid more attention to when his fruits and vegetables would be ready. Sensing my impatience, he reminded me not to underestimate the importance of laying a good foundation, even if I couldn't see the benefits directly. What he knew intuitively was that the deeper the roots, the better the yield. In hindsight, I realize how much he understood about attachment. He worked at cultivating strong roots to fuel and sustain growth. He wasn't big on short cuts and contrived means of getting there; he was organic to the core.

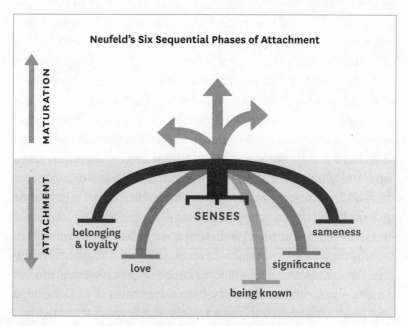

Figure 4.1 Adapted from Neufeld *Attachment Puzzle* course

Neufeld's Six Sequential Phases of Attachment detail how attachment ideally unfolds over the first six years of life. Each sequential phase should add greater complexity and depth to a child's capacity to attach to others. Each phase should deliver a new form of pursuing someone and being able to hold them close. The more ways a child can keep their attachments close, the greater the fuel for their growth into separate, adaptive, and social beings. Although children are born with the capacity for relationship, their attachment instincts need to be activated by consistent and predictable care. It is never too late for attachment potential to be realized, even if it didn't unfold in the first six years of life.

1. **Attaching through the Senses—At Birth**

In the first year of life, children are sensory beings, awakening to their external world and attaching through touch, taste, smell, hearing, and seeing. They may reach to touch hair or faces and give wet gummy kisses, as if trying to devour people. Many babies want to be held close, with their eyes searching for caretakers and with shrieks of alarm ensuing when they are no longer in visual contact. The soothing power of a lullaby stems from a baby feeling close when hearing a familiar voice. Babies also start to make sounds aimed at their caretakers, including coos, babbles, and name-calling—"dada," "mama." They are tuned in to familiar smells associated with loved ones, such as Mommy's perfume: if their attachments are out of sight and sound, they can still be in "smell." A child's overall sensitivity and sensory receptiveness will shape the type of interactions they find soothing.

Consistent and regular physical contact with caretakers is needed to build attachment at the senses level. Although babies are primed at birth to recognize the sounds and smells of their biological mother, it takes 6 to 8 months on average for their brains to be developed enough to lock on to one person as a primary attachment figure.[10] This can also develop later than the 6- to 8-month period if separation resulted from environmental factors. The beautiful design of attachment is such that a primary attachment isn't necessarily to the person a child is born to but rather to the person who consistently cares for them. Children are inclined to attach to the people who offer them the best invitation and consistency of care. This primary attachment will be key in shaping the child's early identity and in unfolding their capacity as a relational being. This person will also be able to introduce the child to other attachment figures, building the village that will help raise them.

2. **Attaching through Sameness—Age 1+**

If all is unfolding well, the one-year-old child will start to hold on to their attachments through imitation and mimicking. They are natural copy-cats, and assume the sounds, preferences, and mannerisms of those they are attaching to. In short, being the "same as" someone is a means of holding them close. A mother of a two-year-old named Jamie relayed the following conversation between her son and his grandmother over lunch one day:

> Jamie: "Nana, have mine."
> Grandmother: "It's okay, Jamie. I have my sandwich. You eat yours."
> Jamie: "No, Nana, please."
> Grandmother: "Really, Jamie, Nana is okay. I don't like bacon. Nana just eats vegetables."
> Jamie: (Looking upset) "Nana, please eat bacon."
> Grandmother: "I am sorry, sweetie, Nana doesn't like it."
> Jamie: (Starting to cry) "Oh, Nana, please like bacon. I like bacon."

We often remark how children "learn" things from their parents as if it were purely a cognitive task. What is missed is how attachment fuels an emotional need to be the same as people closest to you. Children are *moved by desire* to adopt the same shape and form as their attachments. Attachment fuels the quest to imitate, eat the same food, and acquire language—hence the saying "learning one's mother tongue." The values a child adopts have more to do with to whom they are attached than with the outcome of learning. If their peers have become their closest attachments, they will mimic and copy them, giving rise to immature relating. Although we intuitively know a one-year-old is a copy-cat, we gloss over the significance of who they are trying to stay close to through imitation. If you wanted to determine who a one-year-old is attaching to, you need to consider who they talk or act like. The following conversation with parents of a two-year-old boy revealed a surprising attachment figure in his life:

> Deborah: "Who does your one-year-old talk or act like?"
> Father: "Besides my wife and me, I am not sure. Brayden makes a lot of sounds like drills and hammers and uses a lot of imaginary tools around the house."
> Deborah: "Who uses tools in your house?"
> Father: "Not me. My wife doesn't either."
> Deborah: "Does Brayden have grandparents who do? Does he watch TV shows with characters who use tools?"
> Father: "No, he doesn't. The only thing I can think of is we have had a contractor working on our house for the last year and he uses tools."
> Deborah: "I think Brayden is attached to your contractor."

Both parents laughed with this new realization, commenting that their contractor said Brayden reminded him of his son. Adults often consider attachment through roles and responsibilities, but a child considers attachment through the lens of who has delight, enjoyment, and warmth for them.

Attaching through sameness serves the developmental goal of forming a rudimentary working identity. A one-year-old becomes a collection of the characteristics and mannerisms of the people they are relating to. The form they take is the sum total of their identifications with those attachments. Given their immaturity, they hang on to the ideas of others until they form their own. These affiliations are the seeds of their budding personhood, subject to change with increasing sophistication and individuation. For example, little boys may want to wear nail polish like their older sisters, or little girls may want to shave like their fathers. A mother of two young children said, "My children always ask me if they can have my clothes or my jewellery when they get bigger. They also tell me they want to wear 'clip-clop shoes' like me, and want to get their ears pierced too so that they can wear my earrings." The one-year-old's "copy-cat" means of attaching helps form a beginning identity and answers the question "Who am I?" Who they seek to be like reveals the people they are trying to stay close to and is a way of mitigating separation from them.

3. Attaching through Belonging and Loyalty—Age 2+

Growing two-year-olds will begin to attach to people and things through belonging and loyalty. They will start to display possessiveness and territorial behaviour over people and things, claiming them for themselves. Their desire to possess serves the purpose of keeping someone or something close to avoid separation. Attaching through belonging provides a deeper sense of connection to a home base and fitting in somewhere. They may also express delight when parents move to possess or claim them in an exclusive way, with statements such as "There's my girl" or "There's my boy."

Feelings of possessiveness will arise naturally from attaching through belonging. In fact, this possessiveness signals growth in the child as a relational being. The need to possess and ensuing jealousy in sharing someone are "a healthy, normal thing in small children, something that mean[s] that they love, and that they have already made considerable progress in their journey away from the complete immaturity that they started with."[11] A mother recalled how her daughter's possessiveness and jealousy after she turned three were unleashed towards her brother:

> When Brittany's brother, Ben, left the house with his dad, I turned to her and said I was looking forward to spending time with her alone. Brittany looked at me and said, "Mommy, we need to get a new mommy." I was taken aback but managed to ask her why she

felt a new mommy was necessary. She told me, "I want to get a new mommy and give her to Ben, so I can keep you."

Although the possessiveness of the two- to three-year-old can lead to territorial battles, their desires should also be taken as a compliment to the relationship—they seek to claim only the people and things they are attached to. Sharing is overrated in their opinion, making them averse to parting with toys or their people.

A well-developed two- to three-year-old should start to show signs of loyalty after the appearance of belonging. Loyalty involves staying close to someone by obeying rules, following someone, or taking the same side as someone. Showing support of or being devoted to someone is an expression of loyalty. One father described what it was like for visitors to enter his house with his three-year-old, Isabella, as the host:

> When people enter my house, I hear Isabella tell them to "Take off your shoes—that is not allowed," or "Hang up your jackets." Isabella will tell them not to run in the house and to be nice to her brother even when he is loud and crying. She even takes them for a tour of the garden and tells them all the names of the flowers. People think she is smart, but she just repeats what we do and what she hears us saying.

Loyalty is also commonly expressed in two- to three-year-olds as they start to pick sides in disagreements. One mother relayed the following story that happened in the car as the family was heading out for dinner:

> My husband was driving and we were going out for dinner. I decided to give him some friendly driving instructions and encouraged him to take a short-cut to the restaurant. He didn't like my "back-seat driving" and told me, "I think I can figure out where to

park and how to drive after 20 years of driving." I told him I was just trying to help because the route he was taking was really busy. All of a sudden, Nathan yelled at his father, "Daddy, why don't you just listen to Mommy? She knows where to go."

A young child's loyalty is very personal and is one of the best signs that attachment is unfolding well in a two-year-old. Preschoolers' possessiveness is not an accident but a necessary condition that allows them to venture forth while ensuring their attachments come with them. Attaching through belonging and loyalty counterbalances the separation faced by becoming their own person.

4. Attaching through Significance—Age 3+

At approximately the age of 3, a child should ideally start to move into attaching through significance. At this time they will seek to be special and dear in the eyes of their beholders. They will long for approval, hunger to be seen and heard, and want to matter to the people they are attached to. The invitation for contact and closeness from an attachment figure is like oxygen for a young child, and they seem to stand a little taller and feel more important as a result. I still remember the desire to be significant to my mother—her smile and warmth made my heart feel full for hours. A mother of a three-and-a-half-year-old told the following story revealing her daughter's hunger for significance:

> I picked up Genevieve from preschool and when we were walking home, I told her I had seen a little girl in her class who was so lovely, she had a big smile, and was really enjoying herself. As I talked about this little girl and how special she was, Genevieve started to get upset. I asked her if she knew the little girl's name and she said, "No!" I then told her the little girl I was talking about was her and that I had been watching her from the window. The smile on Genevieve's face was huge as she realized I had been talking about her all along.

Parents can convey significance to a child by giving them their undivided attention, remembering what is important to them, or conveying enjoyment in being with them.

When a child attaches through significance, they become sensitized to signs of being held dear and in high esteem, a sense of mattering, as well as delight from their attachment figures. They watch for what is significant to a parent and may work for their approval in order to meet their own attachment needs. For example, the child may start to seek attention and praise with exclamations of "Look at me" or "Look what I did" to garner significance—an attachment fix. The problem is, there is no true rest when children have to work at getting their attachment needs met. When they have to work at being significant, they are not resting in the care offered by their attachment figure. When they work at being loved, they cannot play and grow, and may become preoccupied with performances of being "good enough" instead of feeling good enough just the way they are. This is why praise can be problematic with young children, as they may start to work to please their caretakers in order to receive significance. A healthy sense of self is built upon feeling lovable as one is, and self-worth should unfold naturally.

A child wanting to be significant to someone will be more vulnerable than in previous phases of attaching. When children seek to matter to someone, rejection or lack of invitation by others can be wounding and alarming. A three-year-old's experience of not being welcomed or wanted can lead to shame, the feeling there is something wrong with who they are. This can lead a child to try to make themselves more appealing in the eyes of their beholder or to diminish who they are to fit into the attachment parameters that are deemed acceptable. For a child's self-esteem to have solid ground, a sense of significance needs to be separated from their performance.

A three- to four-year-old uses their attachment figures as psychological mirrors to reflect their emerging identity. What they see will influence how they come to see themselves, especially with signals that are repetitive and intense in nature. For example, if a child sees that their parent enjoys being around them, they will think better of themselves than if they are repeatedly told they are too much to handle or are problematic. The need to matter to someone is a hunger that will drive them to seek significance wherever they can if the home front does not deliver it—just like Penelope did with me. Children need to rest from working at attachment and to read where there is an invitation from another person for contact and closeness and where there is not.

5. Attaching through Love—Age 4+

If development is unfolding well, the four- to five-year-old will give their heart away to their closest attachments. It is the age of emotional intimacy, when protestations of "I love you more" or proclamations of "I am going to marry everyone in the family" abound. Hearts as the symbol of love may become their new motif, appearing routinely in pictures and projects. A tenderness, a softness, and a deep caring emerge—it is a wonderful time to parent a young child!

Love is the emotion of attachment; it cannot be commanded and must be given spontaneously. If a child believes they are loved because they are good, nice, helpful, or smart, they are enslaved to repeat performances in order to work at meeting their attachment needs. When they attribute being loved to *what they do* instead of *who they are*, they cannot rest. The essence of an unconditional attachment is that it conveys to a child that they are lovable as they are. There were times when I would tell my young children I loved them and they would roll their eyes and reply that they already knew this. When I asked how they knew this, they looked at me with blank faces and said, "I don't know. I just do." I hope they never feel they need to work at being loved.

Attaching through love involves a deeper vulnerability, especially as the tender emotions of fondness, warmth, and caring surface. Any person the child gives their heart to will have the power to wound them emotionally. A child can erupt in frustration and alarm if they believe they are no longer cherished, enjoyed, or cared about, or if their providers show a lack of warmth or affection to them. This is one of the reasons attachment unfolds sequentially: so that four- to five-year-olds are selective in giving their hearts away. They will attach through love only to those they feel a sense of sameness with, belonging to, and significance from; this is nature's way of attaching safely.

Love is a deeper form of attaching that allows a five-year-old to stretch farther away from their home base and try new things. The connection through emotional intimacy exemplifies the exquisite dance between attachment and separation; as children venture forward, they still hold on to a sense of home in their heart.

6. Attaching through Being Known—Age 5+

With ideal development, a five-year-old moves into the final phase of attaching through being known. It is a move towards psychological intimacy, and is one of the most fulfilling forms of relating to another person. At this time a child understands that they can keep their thoughts and feelings concealed, choosing whether to disclose the contents of their consciousness to others. In short, they can keep a secret through their own will. When children attach through being known, it unlocks an inclination to reveal hidden parts of themselves to people with whom they share emotional intimacy. The essence of psychological intimacy is closeness through transparency.

Secrets disconnect a child from their caretaker and stand in the way of deepening intimacy with them. Not being able to express one's feelings and thoughts can lead to a lack of vitality. Humans are wired to share themselves in a vulnerable way. This is not to be confused with broadcasting the self to just anyone, such as the depersonalized attempts to garner "attachment fixes" so prevalent in social media usage today. The need to be known is exclusive to your closest attachments. What fuels it is a yearning to cross the divide that is created with the development of separate consciousness. Psychological intimacy is a hunger for connection of the deepest kind.

Children's inclination to reveal themselves is necessary if parents are to look out for and care for them. This inclination ensures that a child does not conceal important things from them, which is critical well into their adolescent years. One father, puzzled by his daughter's confession one night, made sense of it by understanding her desire to be known by him:

> It was really strange to see Elle with her hand over her mouth as if she was about to burst out with something. Elle was clearly trying to hold something back, but it was like there was too much pressure in her to get it out. I finally asked her what the problem was and she said, "Oh, Daddy, I don't want to tell, but I have to! I hid Oscar's trains on purpose because he wouldn't share them with me."

The bias in Elle to be known by her father was greater than her fear of confessing what she had done wrong. Secrets have the power to separate us from those we want to be known by as well as to bring us closer to them.

Parents are often shocked when their child starts to lie. The good news is, lying demonstrates brain integration and the child's capacity to attend to competing thoughts and feelings. This signals the end of the preschooler personality, but recognition of this sophistication is often lost in the turmoil over lying. At a dinner party someone asked me about her six-year-old son, who had just told his first lie:

> Megan: "Toby looked me right in the eyes and said he didn't take candy out of my purse, but I found wrappers hidden in his room. I was so mad. I took away all of his desserts for a week and told him not to ever lie to me again. What am I supposed to do?"
>
> Deborah: "Oh, Megan, Toby now has the capacity to tell a lie—that is wonderful news! To hear how he can hold two things

together in his head at once—the truth and the lie—this is an amazing developmental feat. I understand you are upset, but do you see what this means?"

Megan: (Looks at another friend, mouth open, eyes bulging) "Is she for real?"

Deborah: "Seriously, Megan, it means his brain has grown out of his preschooler way of seeing the world. You have unlocked the door to so much potential for maturity: he is sophisticated enough to conceal himself from you. He knows lying is not okay—this is not the issue. He didn't want to reveal himself to you—this is the issue. One of the antidotes to lying and sneakiness is a desire to be known by your closest attachments. Does he ever tell you his secrets?"

Megan: "Yes, most of the time—I think?"

Deborah: "Then make it safe for him to do so, even when he blows it. He can now decide who he wants to share his heart with—you need to hold on to your relationship with him in order to make sure it's you."

Megan: "Well, how am I supposed to deal with the fact he has lied to me, then?"

Deborah: "Did you talk to him about why he took the candy? My guess is he wanted candy, knew you would say no, and he didn't want to hear that and couldn't resist the temptation to sneak it. This is what life is all about—he needs to have a relationship with his feelings and impulses that tempt him to take shortcuts and not accept 'no' to the things he wants but can't have."

Megan: "How is this going to stop him from lying again?"

Deborah: "Does he feel sorry about it, and not because you told him to say 'sorry'? You just need to bring this to light so that he can reflect on what he has done and how he feels conflicted about it. This is the message you want internalized—that these impulses and feelings are part of us all—it's how we answer them that is important."

Megan: "Ugh... he won't even talk to me about it now. I have already taken away all of his desserts."

Deborah: "I am pretty sure you will get another chance. The temptation to lie never leaves us."

Not only does the sharing of secrets lead to the fulfillment of attachment needs, but it also promotes growth into personhood. When children reveal themselves to their closest attachment(s), they will come to understand themselves better. Truth telling paves the way for authenticity and integrity in relationships, equipping children for healthy friendships and partnerships later in life. The path to authenticity is paved by adults who support children in revealing themselves in a vulnerable way. Personal integrity is fostered when children have the freedom to share themselves without fear of reprisal and separation. The following conditions are conducive to sharing vulnerable feelings and thoughts:

- A child attaches to the parent first through emotional intimacy in order to unlock the bias to want to be known.

- A child feels safe revealing their vulnerable feelings because it will not lead to separation from their attachments.

- A child receives a warm invitation from a parent to reveal themselves; for example, "You seem to have something on your mind," "You seem kind of grumpy, do you want to tell me about it?" or "Your heart seems sad. Can you tell me about it?"

- The child's expression of feelings and thoughts is facilitated by the parent's reflecting back what they have heard, by empathizing, and by acknowledging them.

THE ULTIMATE GOAL in parenting a young child is to unlock all six forms of attaching in the context of deep, vulnerable relationships with their providers. This can be achieved only if the connection is consistent, predictable, and safe from disruption and if the child can experience their emotions in a vulnerable way. When these conditions are met and a child unfolds as a relational being, their development will be propelled forward.

Attachment fuels growth towards functioning as a separate being—it is a beautiful, paradoxical design. Like dance partners locked in intertwining steps, attachment and separation work in tandem. Children's capacity to stretch towards their human potential is dependent on the depth of the attachment roots that nourish them. As attachment deepens, separate functioning is propelled forward in the opposite direction. Children can venture forth to play only when they are assured of a home base to return to. Attachment is one of the greatest forces in human nature, one that pulls us towards each other. At the same time, it is counterbalanced by forces that push our children towards separate functioning and personhood. It is a perfect union of opposing forces: as we hold on to our children, they are free to play and grow, ultimately becoming separate beings.

How to Foster a Strong Attachment through the Collecting Ritual

ALTHOUGH CHILDREN ARE born with instincts to attach, adults must take an active role in engaging this capacity. One of the most basic ways to convey a desire to be close is through the collecting ritual. We need to invite our children into relationship by collecting their attachment instincts—we need to work at getting their attention. By engaging in the collecting dance, we move into their space in a friendly way and work to get a smile, their eye contact, or perhaps a nod in agreement. For example, you might say, "I see you are building a tall tower with your blocks—that is high! I love blocks too." When they seem receptive to our attention, we can engage them further, providing a touch of contact and closeness. If the child seems receptive, we may choose to continue the conversation or invite the child to share their ideas: "How big are you going to be able to make it? Can I help?"

Although the collecting ritual may seem benign, it is a powerful and natural way of communicating the desire to be close to someone. Our expression of delight, enjoyment, and warmth puts us front and centre in a child's attention and positions us to care for them. The collecting ritual is the continuous representation of the adult as the answer to a child's hunger for contact and closeness, forging and strengthening the relational bond between them. As Benjamin Spock summed it up, if there were one prescription for taking care of a child, it would be to enjoy them.[12]

There is no right way to collect a child; collecting is informed by cultural practices as much as by individual disposition. Some children will be collected through the sound of someone's voice, whereas others prefer touch or eye contact. Examples of collecting vary according to setting and from adult to adult, but there is no shortage of ideas for simply getting in a child's face in a friendly way. What is important to remember is that collecting a child has less to do with strategy or procedure than with a genuine desire to be

PROVIDING A TOUCH OF CONTACT AND CLOSENESS FOR THE CHILD TO HOLD ON TO

- a sign of belonging or something special that belongs to us
- a likeness or similarity, something held in common
- a touch of loyalty and a sign that we stand up for them
- a sign of significance, something beyond the expectations of role relationship
- a touch of warmth or delight, something that suggests liking
- a sign that we truly "get them" in ways that others may not
- some sign that they are welcomed into our presence

Figure 4.2 Adapted from Neufeld *Attachment Puzzle* course

close. I still remember the wonderful way my grandfather would collect me when we visited. He would wait for us on the driveway, and had a big smile on his face as we pulled up to his house. I remember how his blue eyes seemed to twinkle as they looked at me—it felt like I was loved to the core. He welcomed us into his home with food, drinks, and laughter. He collected us because he loved us, not because he had to or was instructed to by a book. He embodied delight, warmth, and enjoyment, and I found myself swept up in wanting to be around him.

One of the most common mistakes made with young children is expecting them to follow orders when they have not been collected. By collecting a child, you are getting them to focus their attention on you and follow you because of attachment instincts. With young children we need to *collect their attachment instincts before we direct them.* Given that they attend to only one thing at a time, pulling them away from playing, getting them to come inside, and other transitions are aided by collecting them first. If you are not front and centre in their focus, you are not in their field of influence.

A mother came to me after a presentation on young children and said, "But it takes energy and time to collect them, and I don't have this in the morning." I asked her how her mornings were working out and she said, "Terrible—we fight every day to get out the door. I have to drop my older child off to school and then the younger one to preschool. I am always running late and exhausted by the time I drop them off. The only thing that works in getting them moving is to give them technology time if they get everything done, but then I can't get them off the devices to leave. Mornings are always a battle." I asked her if her children followed her at other times and she said yes but highlighted the pressured time in the morning as being the most problematic. I suggested she try collecting her kids in the morning and set up some predictable ritual to engage them; for example, read a story, tell them the plan for the day, feed them— just get in their face in a friendly way. I conveyed that it was hard to compete for a child's attention when they were on a device, so perhaps devices could be saved for another time of the day. What was most important in turning things around was being able to show warmth, delight, and enjoyment to her kids in the morning. She said, "But I am worried they won't get ready and I will be late and I am going to have to work at collecting them." I replied, "It sounds like you are already late and working hard at battling them. My guess is, things are unlikely to change unless you lead the way through this. I am not saying you need to work harder but differently. Could you give yourself some room to experiment with collecting your kids in the morning and doing things differently?" She told me she would try and report back. The next day she told me, "I tried collecting them this morning and I couldn't believe it, it actually worked. We had such a wonderful morning!" Her eyes then filled with tears and she said, "I can't believe it. I have been fighting with them so long and this is what I needed to do. I have to admit, I doubted this would work, but now that it has I feel I have my kids back."

What was remarkable was this mother's capacity to use the collecting ritual to turn her morning around so quickly. My guess is she had more power as a parent than she realized. She had probably worked hard to cultivate a relationship with her children but didn't know how to harness the benefits of it. This mother reminded me to never underestimate the force of attachment to pull a child back into orbit around a parent. It underscores *who* is meant to feed children relationally, *how* they need to be fed, and *why* it is so important. The collecting ritual provides all the necessary ingredients for answering our children's hunger for connection.

Peers as Competing Attachments

ONE OF THE most prevalent attachment problems in early childhood today is the phenomenon of peer orientation. *Peer orientation* is the term given for the transfer of a child's attachment needs to their peers over their adults. It is the thesis of Gordon Neufeld and Gabor Maté's book, *Hold On to Your Kids: Why Parents Need to Matter More Than Peers*. When children are peer oriented, they will pursue and prefer their friends when it comes to filling their relational needs. This creates competing attachments between their adults and peers as to who will hold the child's heart closest and thereby lead them. Neufeld and Maté state, "Peer-oriented kids often act, especially around one another, as if they don't have parents. Parents are neither acknowledged nor discussed… Children are not disloyal to us on purpose, they are simply following their instincts—instincts that have become subverted for reasons far beyond their control."[13]

Young children are particularly prone to peer orienting because their immaturity and lack of separate functioning mean they consistently seek contact and closeness with someone or something. The similarity and availability of peers in preschool and daycare settings make them natural substitutes for a child's unmet attachment pursuit. If the adults who care for young children do not actively cultivate relationships with them, they cannot satiate their hunger for connection, leaving the children to seek alternative sources.

The problem with peer orientation is that friends are a poor substitute for adult connection. Their immaturity makes them prone to outbursts and to playing fickle, and they are unreliable when it comes to contact and closeness. Peer orientation can give rise to a number of behavioural and learning problems, such as a lack of respect and deference for adults that care for a child; a clear preference for being with peers and frustration when attempts to connect with peers are thwarted; not following, attending to, or sharing values with their adults; and not seeking their adults out when they need help. Peer-oriented children may also adopt the same mannerisms as their peers in a quest to keep close, thereby suffocating their own individuality. They can suffer from anxiety and can seem less confident overall. There is a difference between having friends and relying on them to fill one's hunger for contact and closeness.

The learning and behavioural problems that stem from peer orientation are evident in a letter shared with me by the father of a four-year-old named Peter. Peter's daycare workers had grown frustrated with his lack of listening and his behaviour in class:

> Peter demonstrates a lack of respect for other children and his care providers. For example, today, when Ms. Mavis was singing a song to the children at circle time, Peter said in a taunting tone to the person next to him, "Why does she always sing in that voice? She always sings so bad like that, right?" followed by laughter. He also said to a friend sitting beside him, about another child who could hear him, "Isn't Noah terrible?" Peter is routinely taunting in his comments and tries to get other children to follow along with him. His behaviour is disruptive to the daycare environment. We have told him these actions are inappropriate but he doesn't seem to listen or even let us come close to him.

After discussing Peter's behaviour at home and in daycare, it became clear that he had become peer oriented. As a result, both of his parents along with his child care providers started to work hard to cultivate deeper relationships with him. They reduced peer contact, collected Peter routinely, took a strong lead by reading his needs, and provided generously for him, including dates with Mom or Dad. As the adults in Peter's life brought him into relationship with them, he started listening and his "disrespectful" taunting disappeared.

The seeds of peer orienting are sown in the early years when adults do not actively collect young children and cultivate deep relationships with them. Penelope, the child who pursued me at the playground, would be at high risk for peer orientation. She was seeking connection wherever she could find it, and if her peers were to become the answer to these needs, her adults would experience a greater loss of influence and direction. They would be diminished in their capacity to take care of her both physically and emotionally. The long-term impact of peer orientation on development can include a host of learning and behavioural problems in the home and at school, as well as potentially tragic consequences as children head into adolescence. Peer orientation contributes to emotional and mental health disturbances, including addiction in adolescence.[14]

Young children need to attach to the adults who are responsible for them. It is a child's pursuit of their parent, teacher, or care provider that empowers that adult in their caretaking role. As Gordon Neufeld and Gabor Maté write, "Who is to raise our kids? The resounding answer, the only answer compatible with nature, is that we—the parents and other adults concerned with the care of children—must be their guides, their nurturers, and their models. We need to hold on to them until our work is done."[15]

Who's in Charge?
The Dance of Attachment

And we are put on earth a little space,
That we may learn to bear the beams of love.
WILLIAM BLAKE[1]

NANCY CONSULTED ME regarding her five-year-old twins, James and Sarah, who had "taken over the house." Nancy and her husband lived from one incident to the next, "walking on egg-shells," waiting for frustration to erupt when they said "no" or for resistance to mount when they gave directions. The kids tried to discipline the parents when "they messed up," giving them time-outs and consequences. The tables had turned, and it wasn't because of a lack of parental love, willingness, or desire to be in charge. The parents were exhausted and the twins insatiable; everyone was anxious. Friends had advised Nancy to come down harder on the twins to "show them who was boss," but this had backfired and led to explosions of negative behaviour. A behaviour-focused counsellor gave Nancy a reward chart to reinforce James and Sarah when they listened and obeyed. The chart worked at first... until the twins turned it around and said they would reward Nancy when she was a "good mother." None of the parenting strategies were effective—Nancy's tricks, treats, consequences, punishments, and coercion continued to reveal her impotence as a parent. She was trying to lead with contrived means of behaviour control. Nothing would change in the house until she addressed *why* her kids didn't follow her. She needed to reclaim her alpha position and change the *instincts and emotions* driving her children's behaviour.

In our first appointment, we discussed the reasons for James and Sarah's move to take charge, as well as the challenges that came with their constant resistance, frustration, anxiety, and commanding demeanour. We discussed how her children were displacing her alpha position and how she needed to regain it if she was going to bring them to rest in her care. We talked about what it means to have an alpha presence, as well as about strategies aimed at conveying to the twins they could trust in her caretaking. We discussed how screaming, yelling, time-outs, and "counting to three" type responses were desperate measures and revealed her powerlessness. Her children were consulted on too many matters, so Nancy was encouraged to seize the lead and read her twins' needs without asking questions. After revealing that she had told James and Sarah she was "seeking help to learn how to take care of them," I suggested she conceal this and convey that she already knew what to do.

Two weeks later, Nancy came back and said she had gone home from our first session to find James and Sarah jumping on the bed, with her husband screaming at them to stop. The kids were ignoring him, but when she entered the room, she stood silently, watching them, her feet firmly planted, her eyes conveying that she was in charge, and her arms crossed. The twins looked at her and stopped jumping, stunned by her demeanour, and said, "Mama?" She replied, "Do we really think we are going to jump on the bed tonight?" Having captured their attention, she said, "Storytime," and went to lead them out of the bedroom. In the corner of her eye she caught her husband trying to imitate her stance, with his arms crossed and eyes focused on the kids. She asked him, "What are you doing?" He replied, "I am copying you. That was really good. What do you call that technique?" Nancy replied, "I call it being in charge." And with that, she led James and Sarah to bed.

The Hierarchical Dance of Attachment

RELATIONSHIPS BETWEEN ADULTS and children need to be *hierarchical* for a fulfilling attachment dance to unfold—the parent needs to lead, and the child needs to follow. This dance is an *instinctive* one that cannot be commanded. It is activated when a parent assumes a caretaking stance and creates the conditions for a child to depend on them. The ultimate purpose of attachment is *to foster dependence of the immature on those responsible for them.* Adults need to inspire and invite young children to depend by seizing the lead in the relationship dance, reading the child's needs, and providing generously for them. Relationships with children were never meant to be equal or based on friendship; they are about assuming responsibility for leading them to maturity.

Children don't just need to be attached to adults, they need to be in right relationship with them. A *right relationship* is one in which a young child accepts the adult as their caretaker and follows their lead. A child needs to rest in the care of the adult rather than tell the adult how to care for them. Nancy's twins were attached to her but were not in right relationship—they were trying to be in charge. As one father asked me, "Why does any child follow their parent?" The short answer is because the parent leads the child through the beautiful combination of *caring* and *responsibility taking*.

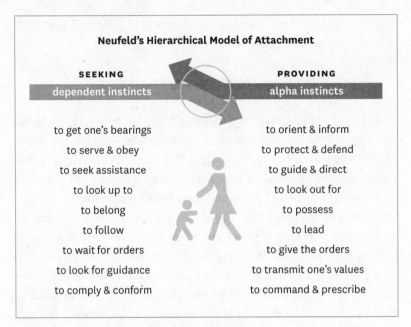

Figure 5.1 Taken from Neufeld *Alpha Children* course

Right relationships are dancelike in nature, with steps governed by innate human drives and instincts. There are two sets of instincts that drive attachment: (1) *alpha instincts*—to assume responsibility for caretaking, and (2) *dependency instincts*—to seek and receive care. Alpha instincts should guide a parent to assume responsibility for providing for a child, and dependency instincts should lead a child to trust their caretaker. When an adult moves into the *provider role*, this should activate a child's instincts to adopt a *seeker role*. This is how attachment becomes synchronous and dancelike. Both parent and child should take their cues from each other and position themselves accordingly. Three-year-old Thomas summed it up well when he said, "I'm going to follow you forever, Daddy."

When a child attaches to a parent through *dependent instincts*, they should be moved to trust, get their bearings, be taken care of, serve and obey, and express their needs, as well as to look for guidance from the adult. It is attaching in a dependent way that naturally moves a young child to comply with adult commands. Parents complain when a young child doesn't listen and obey, as if the deficit lies in the child. What isn't questioned is whether a young child is attached to the parent and is moved to follow them.

Young children are not designed to obey people they are not attached to; this is nature's way of preserving the lead of their attachment figures. However, young children are routinely put in situations in which they are expected to follow commands without a pre-existing relationship; for example, in drop-in programs, with new teachers or care providers, or in the context of dental or medical appointments. The mother of five-year-old Sophia said her daughter spoke rudely to a parent she didn't know at the park. The parent had ordered her to do something, but Sophia wheeled around and said, "You're not my mother. You can't tell me what to do!" The fault lies not in Sophia but in expectations that she take orders indiscriminately. Consequently, the first order of business when taking care of a young child is to build a relationship to foster dependency. It is right relationships that open their ears and hearts to influence, not a caretaker's title, educational degrees, legal rights, or authority over them.

Alpha instincts help steer a parent towards assuming the driver's seat in a child's life. The activation of alpha instincts brings with it a weighty sense of accountability, as well as guilt when mistakes are made. There is an increased sense of alarm and protectiveness, giving rise to "mother bear" or "father bear" type responses, along with deep caring that makes sacrifice possible. When an adult assumes the provider role, their alpha instincts should move them to defend, direct, look out for, possess, give orders to, and share their values with a child. Parents often tell young children, "This is the plan for the day," as they move to orient, inform, and give orders. Alpha instincts should move a parent to hide their own needs so that a young child isn't made to feel responsible for their emotions, stress, hardships, and sacrifices. Young children shouldn't work at taking care of their parents but should rest in their parents' caretaking.

Young children instinctively pay attention to the hierarchy in relationships because this is how they order their world and find their place in it. Four-year-old Fiona explained it to me this way: "I am the boss of my little sister and Mama is the boss of me. Mama is the boss of Daddy, too." What is important to consider is how the young child interprets the hierarchy, which will not necessarily reflect how society construes authority and roles. A teacher, parent, or child care provider may have the title and responsibility of being in charge, but unless the child's instincts perceive them as being in the alpha position over them, the child's dependency will not be activated. The hierarchical ordering of human relationships is what gives a young child a sense of predictability, stability, and faith that they will be cared for.

Sensitive or "orchid" children can be more challenging to bring into right relationship because depending on another person is a vulnerable place to be. They are typically more perceptive and affected by signs that a caretaker doesn't know what to do with them or that they are too much or too difficult to manage. To bring a sensitive child into right relationship requires a strong, safe, and generous provision of care by an alpha adult. It is important to give them time to accept the relationship and to feel comfortable, as many sensitive kids do not respond well to pushing.

The secret power of attachment lies in how it moves us into right relationship with each other. It is a synchronous, reciprocally fuelled hierarchical dance: the more an adult provides, the more a child should rest in their care; the more a child depends on an adult, the easier it is to provide for them. What matters is how this relationship becomes internalized and leads to an exclusive and personalized experience. When right relationships are formed, they cannot be easily replicated or competed with, as they are fulfilling to both parties.

The Alpha Child and the Failure to Depend

A PREVALENT ATTACHMENT problem in early childhood today (in addition to peer orientation, discussed in chapter 4) is that of the alpha child.[2] Alpha problems arise in children when the natural attachment hierarchy becomes inverted; that is, when a child moves into the alpha position instead of staying in a dependent one with their adults. An alpha child is instinctively and emotionally driven to dominate an adult when they no longer feel secure depending on them to be in charge of their caretaking. Instead of following an adult, they command others, telling them what they need and how to care for them. Instead of obeying an adult, the alpha child expects the parent to defer to their wishes and demands. They orchestrate interactions with their adults, even feigning helplessness to evoke caretaking responses. Alpha children are instinctively driven to see themselves as in charge, moving to displace their parents' alpha role.

The alpha problem is *not a learned one* and is meant to serve a child's emotional needs, as it offers them a greater opportunity to be cared for. This was the problem with Nancy's twins, James and Sarah—they had moved into the alpha position in relationship to their parents. The problem was not in the twins but in the lack of right relationship with their adults. They no longer trusted in the caretaking they were receiving at home. Being dependent on another person is a vulnerable place and requires trust. For an alpha child the vulnerability of dependence is too alarming, and as a result, their brain instinctively moves them into the alpha position so as to ensure emotional survival. The problem is you cannot take care of a child who does not depend upon you.

Each alpha child can behave differently, but caretaking often feels difficult, if not a nightmare. Parents often describe their alpha child as insatiable and unmanageable. Instead of following their adults, they can be full of commands, telling their adults, "You're not in charge of me. I tell you what to do." This is not to be confused with a three-year-old who will sometimes exclaim, "You're not the boss of me," or "I do it myself." The alpha problem arises from a deep-seated lack of dependence, with its characteristics being more chronic instead of fluid and variable. The alpha child is often misperceived as being strong and independent, masking the desperation underneath. They have lost faith in their providers to take care of them, so their instinctive recourse is to do it themselves.

Young children who get stuck in the alpha position are quick to *resist and oppose* requests made of them because it doesn't feel right to follow and depend on others. Alpha children display *high levels of frustration* because their adult relationships aren't fulfilling, and may become aggressive when thwarted in their demands. For example, Nancy's twins' frustration spilled over into peer relationships, leading to fights and altercations. Alpha children may have *alarm problems*, including anxiety and agitation, because they do not feel safe and cared for. James and Sarah both displayed anxiety, which affected their ability to pay attention and interfered with learning at school. They can exhibit *eating problems* because being fed activates dependency instincts, which are being defended against. James refused to

COMMON CHARACTERISTICS OF ALPHA CHILDREN

- can be bossy, controlling, or demanding, even when with one's equals or with those one should be depending upon
- seeks to be on top or take centre stage all the time
- can be compelled to take over or to take charge in situations where this is not called for
- can be driven to show superiority with one's equals
- can have difficulty taking direction or asking for assistance
- driven to trump interaction or to have the last word, even when with one's equals or with those one should be depending upon
- must be in the know all the time / can act as a know-it-all

Figure 5.2 Adapted from Neufeld *Alpha Children* course

eat at the dinner table, and Sarah commanded her mother to make certain types of foods every evening.

When alpha problems arise, young children will morph into restless hunters with little freedom to play and grow into personhood. As one parent described the situation,

> Logan doesn't seem happy and is frustrated a lot of the time. He can't play on his own and demands I play with him. He gets mad when I don't do exactly what he wants. Even when I spend a whole day with him, he gets upset when I have other things to do. Nothing is ever good enough and he just seems to have all this energy to burn. Even after playing hockey, riding his bike, going to the park, he is just wired at night—he doesn't seem to ever feel tired.

Logan's father was clearly frustrated, his despair and exhaustion palpable. When he started to understand the alpha problem underlying Logan's behaviour, he became more hopeful that there was a way through.

The challenge with an alpha child is that their characteristics and problems are interpreted as disconnected clusters of behaviour, detached from the inverted relationship that gives rise to them. Parents and helping professionals can get sidetracked battling symptoms instead of connecting the pieces and unearthing the alpha issue. As one psychiatrist exclaimed when I explained the alpha child phenomenon, "I have medicated these kids, and I don't even like to medicate children!" An alpha child usually comes across as strong and independent, blinding us to the desperation beneath their bravado. They don't appear needy and are resistant to being helped by the people closest to them. Furthermore, their behaviour does little to draw out alpha caring instincts in adults because it can be so alienating. The good news is, when you understand the nature of an alpha problem, you can strategically move to unmake it. When an adult regains the lead in the attachment dance, a child will be free to depend, leading them to rest, play, and grow again.

Why Are We Giving Rise to Alpha Children?

WHAT ISN'T GENERALLY well understood when it comes to attachment is that feeling loved by a parent isn't enough; a child needs to feel taken care of and believe that care will endure. A young child needs to feel there is something solid in their parent that they can lean against and count on. If not, they may instinctively move to be in charge of the relationship and become preoccupied with getting their attachment needs met.

There are obvious reasons why a young child may lose faith in their adults—parental neglect, self-absorption, or addiction. However, alpha issues are also found in loving and caring homes, with parents who are dedicated to helping young childen grow to be socially and emotionally responsible individuals—just like Nancy. What is contributing to the dismantling of the natural attachment hierarchy between parents and children today?

One of the biggest challenges faced by parents of young children is the lack of cultural support for their role as an alpha caretaker. When the answers to raising a child are contained in books instead of in parents themselves, we are neither empowering parents in their role nor supporting them in getting into the driver's seat. When there is pressure to get a young child to grow up faster, parenting practices are pushed into the realm of competitive sports instead of supporting values such as patience, time, and faith that a developmental agenda will deliver maturity. When parents resort to measuring progress by counting the number of activities their child engages in, their proficiency with technological devices, or their academic achievements, the answer to growth is detached from the parent–child relationship. When children are pushed to be independent too soon, they will take the lead out of necessity.

Unfortunately, many popular caretaking practices today contribute to the alpha phenomenon because they invert the parent–child relationship. There are seven practices in particular that foster alpha problems.

1. **Parents' Reactions to Their Own Background**

When the type of caretaking a child receives is based on a parent's reaction to their own background, it does little to provide for the needs of the child. For example, if a parent had an authoritarian parent, they may react by being too permissive in order to avoid inflicting the same wounds on their child. It is the parent's feelings that are being cared for in this situation rather than the child's need to have limits and restrictions enforced in a compassionate way. In another scenario, if a parent had little support for their tears and sadness growing up, they may struggle to help their child face limits and restrictions because it creates upset they are uncomfortable with. A mother told me,

> It's hard to watch my child cry and be sad about the things I say no to. As a child I wasn't allowed to be unhappy about anything. The goal was to think positive and to see the glass as half full. I was made to feel bad when I was sad, as if there was something wrong with me. I struggle with these feelings every time I have to set limits and give my child room to feel frustrated, sad, or upset. The good news is the more I understand why this is important for her, the more I am able to do it.

If caretaking is steered by an adult's unmet needs or in reaction to their background, this can displace natural parental alpha instincts and move a child to take charge.

The remedy for adults is to aim for reflection and transparency when it comes to their personal expectations and motivations. We can start by reflecting on what works or doesn't work for our child, focus on making sense of their needs, ask for feedback from an adult when a different perspective is needed, and form intentions for how to show up for our child each day.

2. Parenting on Demand

The alpha caretaker role is an active one in which the parent seizes the lead by assuming responsibility for reading the needs of a child and providing generously. If a parent takes a passive approach to caretaking and simply meets a child's demands, they will place a child in a position of responsibility for getting their needs met. For example, if a child says, "I am hungry. I need something to eat," a parent has missed the opportunity to read their needs and provide for them. Sometimes parents are too busy or exhausted, or they discover they are not interested in some of the responsibilities associated with their caretaking role. Nonetheless, if they do not seize the lead, they can create the conditions for a young child to move into a position of dominance in their relationship.

3. Egalitarian Parenting

Young children can be consulted on too many matters about their caretaking. Questions such as "What do you want to eat?" "Do you want a sleepover?" "Do you want to see your grandparents or go on an outing?" "Which child care provider do you prefer?" and "What school do you want to attend?" suggest that a child has authority when they should not. When children are put in charge of matters concerning contact and closeness with attachments or about their caretaking, this will court alpha problems.

A young child needs to take for granted that they will be cared for, not turned into a consultant regarding their needs. This isn't to suggest that a young child shouldn't be given choices, rather that these choices shouldn't be about caretaking matters, such as food, safety, or contact and closeness with their attachment figures. Choices about what pants they want to wear, which bedtime story they desire, or which toys they want to play with provide them with wiggle room to stretch and flex their growth into a separate being.

Parents of a five-year-old alpha child named Monica were struggling. The problems stemmed partly from her father's approach of not saying no and asking too many questions regarding caretaking matters. I asked the parents if the mother could go out one night a week and leave the father in charge. The two things I hoped he would experience were (1) saying no when needed while being compassionate if Monica was upset and (2) not asking caretaking questions and leading the interactions throughout dinnertime, bathtime, and bedtime. The father was agreeable and welcomed the opportunity to care for Monica on his own. On the first night, the mother received a crisis call within two hours from Monica, who was upset. She said, "Mama, you need to come home. I don't know what happened to Daddy, he said 'no' to me and is talking all funny. Can you come home and fix him?" The mother reassured her that Daddy knew exactly what he was doing and she was fine in his care. As Monica's mother stepped out each week, her father stepped in to take on a more alpha role, and Monica's dominance problems diminished.

4. Too Much Separation

Separation anxiety is prevalent among young children and reflects their irreducible need for attachment. Although physical separation is part of a young child's daily experience, too much of it, or a connection that is unreliable or inconsistent, can invert the adult–child relationship. When a teacher or child care provider cares for a young child, right relationships need to be developed to prevent the child from moving into an alpha stance. Although adults may consider child care to be a paid service, children will be receptive to being cared for only if they have strong parental substitutes to rely on. Child care providers tell me they know when a child is finally feeling at home with them when that child calls them Mom or Dad "by mistake."

One day a mother called me in distress when a preschool teacher had punished her daughter by taking away her locket that contained a family picture. Emma, age 4, was distraught and no longer wanted to attend the preschool. She refused to ask for help from her teachers and wouldn't eat her lunch or follow directions. The less Emma obeyed, the more time-outs and consequences she received from her teachers, giving rise to an alpha stance with them. Her teachers were unwilling to change and couldn't resuscitate their relationship with Emma. The parents were left with no choice but to switch pre-schools to make headway with the alpha problem.

Emma's story conveys how critical it is for adults to activate a child's instincts to depend. This happens only when a child is assured that caretaking won't expose them to ridicule or separation from people and things they are attached to. When young children are disciplined in ways that leverage their attachment needs and create separation alarm to achieve compliance, it does little to foster strong caretaking relationships. A lengthier discussion on discipline and young children can be found in chapter 10.

5. **Bullying by Parents, Siblings, Peers, or Teachers**
The experience of being wounded emotionally or physically by an adult or another child fuels alpha problems. For example, if a pre-school teacher cannot tame a bully in a class, the class will probably feel unsafe for other children. If a parent doesn't move to shield and protect a child from a sibling who bullies, the greatest wound is not from the sibling but from the parent's failure to make home safe. It is the violation of protection that has the most impact on a child and creates emotional distress along with alpha problems.

6. **Overwhelming Sensitivity and Extreme Vulnerability**
Some children are born too sensitive for their world, with an enhanced sensory receptiveness leading to feelings, thoughts, and stimuli that overwhelm them. A sensitive child can feel intensely, swinging wildly from passion to despair. Their strong reactions can overwhelm their adults, as reflected in statements from parents such as "You're too much for me!" "Why are you so dramatic?" and "I don't know what to do with you!" Such expressions can undermine

a parent's lead, as they convey that a parent doesn't understand the child or know how to take care of them. Sensitive kids need strong alpha parents who can remain in their caretaking stance despite the tremendous emotions and difficult behaviours that come out of a young child.

7. Alarming Experiences or Circumstances

Alarming experiences and events can overturn right relationships by suggesting that a parent cannot keep their child safe despite their good intentions. I have helped parents get back into the lead after their child has experienced broken bones, car accidents, root canals, surgery, or burglaries, or when someone has died. The good news is, when an adult assumes a strong caretaking stance, a child can rest again in their care, but it often takes time and patience.

Taming an Alpha Child

IF WE FAIL to see the root of an alpha problem in inverted attachment, we can end up attacking the symptoms of resistance or opposition, frustration or aggression, anxiety or agitation, or eating problems in a way that exacerbates the underlying alpha problem. The only lasting solution is for an adult to regain the lead in the attachment dance. The challenge is, everything works in reverse with an alpha child—they listen to people they are not attached to and won't obey the ones they are closest to. Their closest attachments bear the brunt of their worst behaviour and are baffled, as they are usually the ones who care for the child the most. Natural caretaking instincts cannot guide a parent with an alpha child because of the child's lack of dependency on them. There is also the challenge of hearing critical remarks about one's parenting and receiving unsolicited advice. This puts the parent in a dependent role rather than supporting the parent in getting into the driver's seat. Most advice fails to understand the instinctive and emotional roots of the alpha problem.

Given the intense resistance and opposition of the alpha child, along with their frustration and aggression, it is common to hear they need a "harder hand" to teach them a lesson. Alpha problems arise not from failed lessons but from a lack of reliance on a caretaker. If a parent's response is to exploit a child's dependency, remove things, punish, or lord authority over them, they will do little to court reliance. At the same time, a parent cannot give in to demands and fail to lead through the storms that occur. The place a parent must lead an alpha child from is caring dominance—the adult is in charge, and the child will not experience this as adverse or emotionally wounding. It is through warmth, generosity, and being able to set limits while dealing with upset that an adult can convincingly demonstrate they are a child's best bet.

The following eight strategies can assist a parent in regaining the lead in the attachment dance, as well as prevent them from losing their lead. Support from professionals who understand the alpha problem may be sought, as well as additional resources from the Neufeld Institute listed at the back of this book, including the course on Alpha Children.[2]

1. Convey a Strong Alpha Presence

One of the most important strategies for taming an alpha child is to lead by assuming responsibility and conveying an alpha presence. This means you assume responsibility for making headway in righting the relationship, for keeping the child out of harm's way, and for not putting them in situations that are too difficult to manage them in. A parent of an alpha child needs to connect with their own desire to take care of their child and engage with the child from there. The parent may not feel inclined to connect because of the child's behaviour, but it is a critical step forward in unmaking an alpha problem. If a child with an alpha complex sees that they baffle and defy their adult, then they cannot trust in the caretaking offered. An alpha child will get frustrated when someone won't give in to their demands, but the feeling they are too much or are overwhelming will only reinforce their alpha stance. An adult needs to convey that they are the answer the child seeks when it comes to contact, closeness, and being cared for.

2. Make It Easy and Safe for the Child to Depend on You

If they are to lead an alpha child, a parent needs to make it safe to be depended upon. It will be difficult to build a trusting relationship when authority is used to force compliance by taking things away or denying agreed-upon privileges. Adversarial relating caused by the use of time-outs, threats, and consequences will exacerbate a young child's alpha stance. A parent must steer through stormy behaviour and convey that they can manage the situation.

The key strategy with an alpha child is not to appear displaced from one's caretaking stance and not wound them in the interaction or appear passive in one's response. When Nancy began to sidestep battles with her twins and refused to negotiate with them as if they were equals, she started to change the tone in the house. For example, when Sarah took away James's toy and hit him, Nancy took charge by saying, "Brothers aren't for yelling and hitting, Sarah. I am going to hold on to the toys right now and I will talk to you both about it later. We are going to do something different now." She would sometimes circle back to the incident later in the day or in a moment of privacy with each child. She would acknowledge their feelings of upset and, if they seemed amenable, give them directions for handling similar situations in the future.

Most incidents are better dealt with outside the moments they occur, but sometimes a parent's hand is forced. At these times, it is necessary to maintain an alpha caring stance and ride out the storm. For example, one mother said her three-and-a-half-year-old son would battle her on everything, but especially on wearing a jacket when it was cold outside. She decided to wait her son out by letting him know they would head to the park when the jacket was on.

Dominic screamed and yelled, but Mom stayed calm and told him she knew this would happen. After screaming for some time, Dominic's brain finally understood that his defiance was futile and his mother wasn't going to change her mind. Although his mother was successful in getting Dominic to wear his jacket, the more important message was that his mother was in charge and it was safe to depend on her.

The key issue in being able to depend on a parent is that a child's neediness, inferiority, smallness, fears, and dependency cannot be taken advantage of. Although finding one's way through tricky situations requires patience and creativity, protecting both the child and the parent's dignity can go a long way in righting inverted relationships.

3. Read the Needs and Take the Lead

One of the challenges with an alpha child is that they make continual demands on their caretakers. You cannot take care of a young child when they are directing you. The goal is to meet their *needs* instead of their *demands*. One strategy is to trump their requests by giving them more than what they ask for. For example, if an alpha child demands that a parent dress them, instead of meeting their request, read their need and trump it: "I was just going to get your pants and socks because I knew you wanted help getting dressed. I even have your favourite jacket ready too." When a parent trumps the child's demands and provides for the underlying need, it communicates that the parent understands them, can be counted upon, and is in charge. For example, Nancy's mornings with James were full of commands and frustration, so she took the lead and got to him first. At some point James said to her, "I don't know what is happening to me. I used to have this yes/no board in my head and every time you wanted me to say yes, the board moved to no. Every time you wanted a no, the board moved to yes. I'm scared, Mommy, my yes/no board is disappearing." As James became less resistant, he was easier to take care of. As Nancy felt more effective as a parent, her confidence to lead James increased. The more her confidence increased, the more inclined James was to follow, restoring their dance of right relationship.

4. Provide a Legitimate Expression for Alpha Instincts

Giving a young child an outlet for their alpha instincts can help reduce the intensity of these instincts in the parent–child relationship. These outlets can be fostered through structured activities or play. For example, Nancy enrolled James in piano classes, which he loved. He started to compete with himself to see how far he could advance, and how fast. Nancy enrolled Sarah in karate, where her competitiveness was vented through a solo sport. Nancy also found that one of Sarah's favourite play activities was setting up a veterinary clinic where she was responsible for saving all of the animals. Sarah bossed her imaginary employees around and instructed everyone on the proper ways to heal wounded animals. She concocted scenarios in which only she could be the one to save the day. In her play, Sarah was able to express her alpha instincts, sparing Nancy the brunt of some of her commands and demands. The key is finding areas young children can be in charge of that don't compete with the caretaking responsibilities of the parent.

5. Foster Natural Hierarchical Relationships

When children are embedded in natural attachment hierarchies, their instincts to depend can be appropriately activated by roles and contexts. For example, Sarah and James had older cousins whom they adored and followed. Their cousins didn't respond to their bossy ways and took a firm lead when it came to doing activities such as sports together. Sarah and James's grandparents, aunts, and uncles were also instrumental in righting the attachment hierarchy, introducing the twins to hobbies, playing games with them, and taking them on outings.

The parents stopped placing Sarah and James in same-age play-dates and focused on their relationship with each child instead. They started separating James and Sarah from each other and spent more time one on one. They looked for opportunities for Sarah and James to be around younger children, so as to draw out their alpha instincts in a healthy, caretaking way. The focus shifted to changing the twins' environment and embedding them in a natural relational hierarchy, rather than trying to change their behaviour. The shift in context served to convey their place in the hierarchy and activate their instincts to depend.

6. Take Charge of Circumstances and Decisions

Leading a child means conveying that you know what they need without consulting them and assuming responsibility for circumstances or decisions about them. For example, one day while shopping, Sarah demanded that her mother buy her a watering can. Nancy told her she would think about it and would let her know once they finished getting groceries. At the end of their trip, Nancy turned to Sarah and said, "I have thought about it and I have decided I would like to buy a watering can for you because you will have fun with it in the garden." Sarah replied that she no longer wanted the watering can, though her teary eyes and buckling lip said otherwise. The mother took the lead and told Sarah she was going to buy it as she knew Sarah would want to play with it later. The challenge for Sarah was that the vulnerability of depending on her mother was too much at this time, and her alpha instincts pushed away her mother's attempt at caretaking. The mother's actions conveyed to Sarah that she was in charge and that it was safe to rely on her.

When dealing with any child, it is also important to hide one's own fears and needs from them, especially when they are stuck in the alpha position. Otherwise, a child will read the parental fears or concerns and possibly move to dominate or care for a parent. Furthermore, telling an alpha child the parenting agenda or strategy for dealing with them will only increase their resistance to it. For example, if a parent says, "You make me feel angry when you scream at me and refuse to do what I say," the screaming and resistance will probably increase. Being explicit with instructions or directions invites a child's alpha instincts to take charge and perform the opposite behaviour as a means of asserting dominance. Less explicit requests will work better, for example, "I wonder what the weather will be like today when we walk to preschool" instead of "Get your jacket on. We are going to school." Although there are probably few parents who wouldn't feel frustrated when their child doesn't obey, the key is to not reveal your impotence.

One of the hardest challenges in dealing with an alpha child is not taking their behaviour personally and not reacting to them out of uncontrolled emotion. Parents can feel exhausted, upset, and hopeless. Sometimes they can't believe how hard parenting has become, may struggle to find their love for their child, and may fight with their partner about how to make headway. It is hard to hang on to hope that right relationships will prevail in the midst of problem behaviour and challenges. A parent needs to take a step back and understand the root of the alpha problem. This will allow them to anticipate the problems, get ahead of those problems, and hold on to the big picture of how they are trying to alter course.

7. Set the Stage for Being the Child's Answer

An effective strategy with an alpha child is to find opportunities when the child must depend upon their parent, including teaching them a hobby or going on an outing. Many alpha children refuse to go out of the house because that is their "kingdom" or because a direct request has been made of them. Despite their protests, leading them to a new place or activity can dislodge their alpha stance, albeit temporarily, and provide the parent with an opportunity to lead. Parents often remark how wonderful their young child is on these outings and how dismayed they are when the alpha characteristics reappear back at home. It takes time to tame the alpha child, and the steps forward are small. As examples of such small steps, Nancy started taking James out to catch frogs, and he was thrilled to have time alone with her and to learn about some of his favourite creatures. Nancy also capitalized on her twins' dependency when they were sick or in trouble. Exhibiting strong caretaking at these times fostered a sense of trust and reliance on her.

When Nancy found the alpha parent inside of her, it was beautiful and breathtaking. She came into my office, telling me how she had steered through tricky situations, what she couldn't make sense of, and where she longed for understanding. Nancy worked to reclaim her rightful place in James's and Sarah's lives by seizing the lead—not through techniques, remembering mantras or directions, or using bribes, threats, or punishments. What she found was much more convincing and would take her their full distance into adolescence. As Nancy's alpha instincts came to life, she activated her twins' dependent instincts and began to pull them into orbit around her. She was surprised it had been inside of her the whole time. As Nancy's husband witnessed her success, he also started coming in for counselling sessions to better understand his children and get into the driver's seat.

We need to dance our way into right relationships with our children by (a) ACCEPTING the WORK of the relationship is our responsibility, (b) ASSUMING an ALPHA role by seizing the lead and reading the child's needs, and (c) PROVIDING more than is pursued so that our provision of care more than satisfies their hunger for connection. There is great dignity and growth for parents in claiming their rightful place in a child's life. From this place they will find the confidence to make sense of their child, the strength to lead them, and the courage to trust that their caretaking is enough. We make ourselves irreplaceable when we dance with our children in right relationships.

Feelings and Hurts
Keeping Children's Hearts Soft

The heart has its reasons which reason knows nothing of.
BLAISE PASCAL[1]

C LAIRE STOOD IN a small photographer's studio in Oaxaca City, Mexico. She looked at the walls adorned with portraits of young children smiling, laughing, crying, frowning, or hiding their faces in shyness. Each child's emotions were laid out in circular fashion around a central picture, taking on the semblance of art. Claire wondered why someone would want to freeze frame tantrums and resistance when most parents are happy to avoid them altogether. She found the owner and asked why he captured young children in these states, and he replied matter-of-factly, "The portraits represent all the emotions and facets of life. Some serious and thoughtful, some happy, some sad. Es la vida—that's life." Claire was struck by his explanation: it felt like he had broken a taboo or some sacred tradition by turning grumpiness into an art form. She wondered who the parents were behind these pictures and how they had come to value their child's emotions—even the messy ones.

The portraits left a lasting impression on Claire. What did these portraits have to tell us about our relationship with children's emotions and the quest for happiness? Why weren't these parents concerned with getting their children to calm down, and why did they celebrate the noise within their children? Claire felt these children were fortunate to have guides who were willing to help them learn a language of the heart. The portraits embodied what every child needs—a guardian for their vulnerable feelings and soft hearts.

The Emotional Lives of Young Children

AS EMOTIONAL CREATURES, young children are predictably unpredictable. They have big emotional worlds but few words to describe them. They are full of emotional energy but have no way to control it. They pick up on the emotions of others but don't understand their own. They have good intentions for their behaviour, but these are lost in the intensity of their emotional experience. They have untempered emotional expression that defies reason. Parents of any tantruming or resisting young child will readily attest to their emotional immaturity. For example, when three-year-old Thomas hit his father in frustration, he was directed to use his words instead. Thomas obeyed and said, "I'm going to pee on you, Daddy."

The good news is that young children are the easiest people to read when it comes to their emotional states. Their bodies radiate happiness or frustration, their giggles exude joy, their feet jump when excited or stomp when mad. How a young child feels is usually on display for everyone to see. The challenge is that emotional expression can be big, intense, loud, messy, chaotic, and most inconveniently timed. Tantrums are unleashed in grocery stores, and resistance appears when in-laws come to visit. Children's emotions appear freely despite daily schedules and parental patience levels. The question is, what do we do with a young child's emotions as they bubble up and burst forth? We can't answer this question without considering what is needed to foster emotional health and maturity. We need to take the uninhibited, rampant, and chaotic emotional expression of the young child through to adolescence and towards emotional maturity in adulthood. We have an emotional marathon ahead of us.

The study of human emotion has been hampered by its invisible and ephemeral nature. The behavioural approach put forth by American psychologist B.F. Skinner treated feelings as nuisance variables to be extinguished through reinforcement schedules and operant conditioning.[2] Skinner's views have had a lasting impact; they drive the current smorgasbord approach to discipline that tries to extinguish and calm a young child's emotions as they erupt and spew forth.

To further complicate matters, rationality and maturity have been equated with a lack of emotional expression, though few neuroscientists would support this idea today. Neuroscientists agree that the human brain has preset, hardwired emotions at birth.[3] This view of emotion exists in stark contrast to the blank slate theory, according to which human behaviour is learned and innate and emotional drivers do not exist. Emotions have a purpose and work to do; they are meant to pack a punch and to move us in a way that aids survival and growth.

Antonio Damasio, a leading neuroscientist, has made it clear that the rational part of the brain is built on top of, and in conjunction with, the brain's emotional centre, or limbic system.[4] New discoveries are paving the way in reconceptualizing the role of emotions, including mapping their neurochemistry, neural pathways, and role in brain integration. Fortunately, neuroscience is revealing the critical role of emotions in healthy growth and development. In *The Healing Power of Emotion* Diana Fosha, Daniel Siegel, and Marion Solomon write, "Hardwired to connect with each other, we do so through our emotions. Our brains, bodies, and minds are inseparable from the emotions that animate them. Emotions are at the nexus of thought and action, of self and other, of person and environment, of biology and culture."[5] In short, emotions are the engine of human development.

What Are Emotions?
....

AN EMOTION IS defined as something that stirs us up and moves us into action. Emotions are something that happen to us rather than something under our conscious control. The brain has its own reasons for activating emotions, despite how irrational they may appear on the surface. We can't argue with emotion as if it were logical—there is a method to its madness, a purpose behind its activation. Monsters appear at bedtime, as most three-year-olds will attest, and there are few explanations that will stop their appearance. One mother gave her three-year-old a dream catcher to take away her nightmares, but her daughter said, "Mama, it's broken—the monsters still come out of my eyes when I'm asleep." Another child took a different approach and told her father, "Monsters don't eat your toes if you wear socks to bed," and "I don't sleep with my hands over my head because the gorillas will come and tickle my armpits." Young children will find "logical" solutions to what disturbs them emotionally.

Emotions create an action potential that propels a child towards getting a need met or a problem fixed. In short, emotions are not

EMOTION IS HOW THE BRAIN MOVES THE CHILD...

... to CAUTION when facing what alarms

... to SEEK TOGETHERNESS when hungry for contact and closeness and connection

... to STOP when encountering futility

... to VENTURE FORTH when home base is secure

... to SHY AWAY from contact with those not attached to

... to CARE about one's attachments

... to RESIST when outside of attachment

... to EMERGE as a separate person when attachment hunger is satiated

Figure 6.1 Taken from Neufeld *Heart Matters: The Science of Emotion* course

problems; they provide the impetus and energy to solve problems. If we want to understand how a child is stirred up, we need to consider how they are moving. If a child runs to a parent for cover, it is likely alarm that has sent them there. Their movement towards exploration and discovery is fuelled by a desire to venture forth and grow. *Emotion is the engine that drives human action; it is what the behavioural paradigm has missed in its effort to quantify and measure human behaviour.* Although emotion may be invisible to the naked eye, we can't deny its existence or its capacity to activate us and drive us. Ask any parent who loves their child deeply—words fail to capture how they are moved to care and sacrifice for them.

Emotions are critical to a child's overall development; they are the engines that drive growth into personhood. Children don't need to be taught how to act mature as much as how to feel the right feelings to get there. They need to be moved to caution, to care, to feel sad when faced with life's futilities, to trust, to have confidence and courage, and to hope. It is their vulnerable feelings, especially those of caring and responsibility, that make them humane and fully human. Soft hearts feel emotions in a vulnerable way and are moved by them.

Five Steps to Emotional Health and Maturity

PARENTS ARE A child's first guide in understanding the impulses, emotions, and stirrings within their emotional system. The goal is to develop their capacity to bring emotions under a system of decision making, intention, and reflection so that they can *begin* to share them responsibly. If development is progressing well, this unfolds with the integration of the brain at 5 to 7 years of age, or 7 to 9 for more sensitive children. Parents need to work at providing the conditions to grow children into emotional maturity instead of commanding them to act emotionally mature.

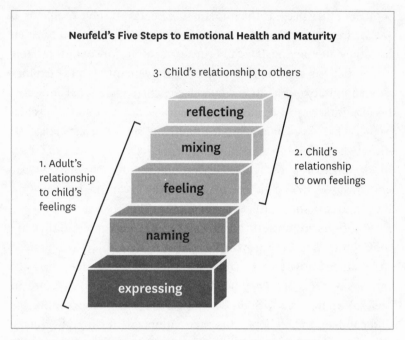

Figure 6.2 Taken from Neufeld *Heart Matters: The Science of Emotion* course

Neufeld's Five Steps to Emotional Health and Maturity involve a sequential development of a child as an emotional being. A child develops a relationship with their emotions over time with the help of adults who introduce the child to their feelings. The five sequential steps cannot be bypassed, and unfold through a series of increasingly sophisticated phases: expressing, naming, feeling, mixing, and reflecting. Parents have three critical roles to play in steering a child through these five steps, shaping their overall potential as emotional beings:

1. Parents are *guides* to facilitate emotional expression and assist a child in learning names for their feelings.

2. Parents are *shields* who preserve soft hearts and assist feelings in becoming conscious.

3. Parents are *tempering agents* who decide how to restore balance and fluidity to a child's emotional system, helping them mix and reflect on their feelings.

1. Parents as Emotional Guides

Emotion seeks expression just like dammed water seeks release. The purpose of emotion is to move a child forward, but it requires a channel to run in and a place to flow. For a young child, the experience of this emotional energy is like being on a river raft heading down whitewater rapids. There is little use in fighting the power of the water, and they cannot help but yield or be swept up by its force. The only recourse is to look for a guide to hang on to and go with them as they cascade over crests, swells, and waterfalls. A young child will need to trust a guide to steer them through tricky parts and deliver them safely to restful waters. The vulnerability of dependence will rear its head often, propelling the child to consider whether a guide can be counted on to care for them. This "emotional ride" is a daily— even hourly—occurrence for young children and their parental guides. The raft is their right relationship, with the adult steering a course forward.

Emotions are supposed to rise up and flow through our children; their existence is not a problem, though they may be the cause of many problems. Parents need to guide a child's emotional system to make sure it remains fluid, open, and vibrant. Parents are naturally positioned to facilitate the expression of a child's emotions and will need to invite those emotions to come forth, as well as provide words to match emotional states. To become a guide, a parent will need to use their own emotional system to understand the emotional state of a child. The capacity to read emotions in others stems from limbic resonance, "the wordless harmony we see everywhere but take for granted—between mother and infant, between a boy and his dog, between lovers holding hands across a restaurant table."[6] A young child should seek emotional refuge in a parent's caretaking; parents are their compass point when they're lost or confused. When a parent can read a child's emotions, invite expression, and communicate that they will care for the child, the right relationship is strengthened. The capacity to read a young child emotionally is how parents become guides and how children learn secondhand about the emotions that exist inside them.

Emotional expression provides the raw material upon which a parent can teach a language of the heart. What is unique about humans compared with other mammal species is we have the ability to give *names* to our emotional states. The name we give to the subjective appraisal of our emotional state is what we call *feelings*. Feelings are the words we consciously use to communicate how we are stirred up. When young children have feeling names for their emotions, their words open the door to greater vulnerability, awareness, and insight. Parents need to invite congruence between a child's heart and mouth, which will be at the root of their integrity and authenticity. When we do not honour what is within a child, we set them on a trajectory to alter themselves to keep us close. We diminish and pollute their selfhood for the sake of taking care of our emotions and all the feelings we cannot handle.

When a child receives an invitation to express their emotions, they also receive the message to trust their heart to provide them with valuable information. As a parent validates a child's feelings, it conveys confidence and faith that their wordless stirrings are to be leaned upon in decision making. When we help our children have a relationship with their feelings, they will be able to share them responsibly with others. Our children need a self to share, a heart that feels, a mouth that tells, and a belief that the richness in life comes from experiencing it in a vulnerable way. When a parent honours a child's emotions, they create expectations for future relationships in terms of emotional and psychological intimacy.

THE PROBLEM WITH INVITING EMOTIONAL EXPRESSION

The problem with inviting a child to express their emotions is that expression can be messy, difficult, crude, chaotic, and uncivilized. How does a parent keep a neutral expression and keep a child's emotions flowing when what is coming out of them is shocking, unacceptable, alienating, and wounding? For example, five-year-old Jasper yelled at his dad, "Take me down to the police station so they can shoot me!" Six-year-old Marina declared to her mother, "Your skin and bones are a waste on your body!" Ethan's mother said that her three-year-old screamed at his father, "I hate you! I want to poke out your eyes and take a chainsaw and chop you into little pieces!" I used this last story as an example with a group of parents one night and was dismayed as they responded with wide eyes, gasps of horror, and exclamations of "How terrible!" I was taken aback because I thought three-year-old Ethan had been quite expressive with his foul frustration, clear with his intentions, and articulate. Where I saw human potential, the parents saw only delinquency.

I was not concerned with Ethan's immaturity; instead, I wanted to understand the reason he had been so stirred up with foul frustration. I asked his mother to tell me the story of what came before his attacking words, and it became clear he was upset because his father had to go to work after being home for some time on vacation. Ethan wanted to play with his dad, and his frustration turned foul when he was told he could not. He chose a chainsaw as his weapon because his favourite activity with his father was to watch him saw wood. What Ethan needed was someone to give his feelings some space for expression and to give him names for what was within his heart. This emotional process and release could be facilitated only by someone he had a good relationship with, who understood his feelings, who acknowledged what was difficult to accept, and who could soften his frustration with warmth. The answer to Ethan's emotions was caretaking. He needed to hear things like "Nothing is working for you right now. You want Daddy to play and he can't," or "You are so frustrated that Daddy has to go to work now." Once Ethan's tears fell, his heart would soften and he would come to accept one of life's hardest truths: sometimes you can't keep the people you love close to you. Why would we want to punish a child for struggling with this? What Ethan wanted was contact and closeness with his dad; what he got was connection with his mother as she guided him to the root of his frustration and finally to his tears.

Parents may struggle to make sense of a young child's emotions, but inviting them to express their feelings doesn't require understanding. At the root of parents' hesitation and fear in giving room for expression is the idea if they "give an inch," a child "will take a mile." Parents fear that the emotional expression will never stop; it will take over and there will be no end to it. Emotional energy doesn't stop until it is released. Dammed-up emotions can create greater eruptions and further explosions. When the emotional system is stirred up, it will continue to press and find a channel for release—anything to reduce the pressure within. Emotions will take more than a mile if you try to press down on them.

Parents can also falsely believe that emotion is learned and must be unlearned with reinforcement and consequences. The new science of emotion has shown that this is incorrect. We do not teach a child to behave frustrated, alarmed, caring, sad—they are born with the capacity to feel these emotions and are instinctively moved from this place. The role of a parent is to guide them through their emotions so that stability, balance, and self-control can eventually be achieved.

The question we need to consider is what would it have meant for Ethan to have been told by his parents, "We aren't going to be around you when you talk like this," or "Go to your room and come out in three minutes," or "You are so mean to your daddy. What kind of a disrespectful boy says things like this?" These words would create an emotional dilemma for Ethan. If expressing the frustration inside of him led to losing the people he wanted most, his brain would enact an intricately orchestrated sacrifice play. Alarm over being separated from his attachments would move his brain to depress or press down on the emotions that threaten his relationships. Like magic, Ethan would appear after his time-out "calmed down" and "good as gold." The alarm created by being sent away would extinguish his frustration and tuck him back into relationship with his parents. The underlying frustration would not be resolved, however; he would still be stirred up, unable to express it, and would have little insight and awareness into it. The cat, the dog, or another child might get the brunt of his frustration, but not his parents, as his brain would strategically move to protect these relationships. Time-outs and separation-based discipline "work" because they hijack the brain's emotional system by creating attachment alarm. If this type of response were enacted often, Ethan would have not only a frustration problem but an alarm one too. Separation is the most powerful of experiences and shapes the emotional brain.

THE PROBLEM OF THWARTED EMOTIONAL EXPRESSION

What does it mean for a child when their brain must suppress emotional expression for the sake of preserving a parental relationship? What is the price to emotional health and maturity when expression is thwarted in a system that was built for movement? The cost is to the relationship they form to their emotions and how they evolve as an emotional being. As a parent responds to a child's emotions, they convey which ones are acceptable, and the landscape of a child's heart is carved into being. If the child desires a relationship with the parent, their brain will unconsciously shape their emotional expression to match the invitation given. Unwelcome emotions are pushed into the darkness, outside of the parameters of what is deemed acceptable, leaving the cookie-cutter outline of their heart to come into view. For example, if a child sees that their father doesn't like it when they are sad and tries to get them to think positively, the child's brain may come to press down on sad feelings in order to make their relationship with Dad work. They may struggle in childhood and into adulthood with their sad feelings if no one else was able to invite their sad feelings and help name them. Thwarted expression can also lead to alpha problems and a host of emotional problems. It is a perfect recipe for depression.

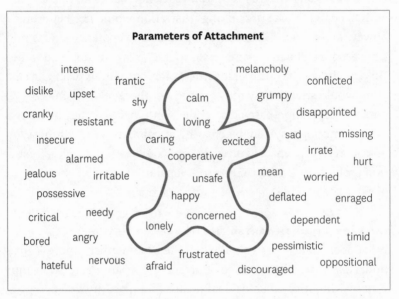

Figure 6.3 Taken from Neufeld *Heart Matters: The Science of Emotion* course

The ultimate sacrifice that results from thwarted expression is in the integrity of a child's inner world and to the sense of vitality that comes from being able to express vulnerable feelings. When a parent conveys warmth and a desire to be close only when a child conforms to the image that pleases them, there is no rest to be found in their caretaking relationship. What is set in motion is a preoccupation with one's performance. A child's spirit becomes crushed, diminished, and defined under the weight of societal and parental needs to behave appropriately. For example, six-year-old Zoe came home after school one day and said her teacher had called her sweet for being so helpful in class. Zoe said, "I love Ms. Lusik. I am going to be sweet for her all the time." Fortunately, her mother understood the need to have a big invitation for all of her feelings and replied, "If you are going to be that sweet at school, then you will need to be extra grumpy at home because no one can be that nice for that long!" The mother wanted Zoe to see that their relationship could take the weight of whatever emotions she might need to express.

The antidote to thwarted expression is conveying to a child that all of their emotions are welcome and won't lead to separation. For example, a young boy watched his mother as she dealt with a tantrum in his older sister. He asked his mother, "Aren't you glad you only have one child like that?" The mother courageously replied, "I could have 100 screaming children and take care of them all. If you need to have a tantrum, you can go for it too." She said he didn't take her up on the offer, but she was happy for the opportunity to convey that she could take care of his frustration too.

Children need a generous invitation to express their heart's contents. The messy parts, the chaotic parts, the hurtful, wounding parts—they are all part of our children too. We have a responsibility to invite all of these into existence, not just the parts we like. How will our children have a relationship with the most "unacceptable" sides of themselves if we cannot lead them there? How do we become guardians of their hearts when we cannot look at their emotions or our own? How can we lead them to civilized and responsible ways of sharing their feelings if we don't allow them to express them? The most powerful message we could deliver is that our relationship can take the weight of who they are and whatever comes out of them. In the moments they are full of wounding words, chaos, and emotional disorder, we need to offer an invitation for connection that can bridge whatever comes between us.

Young children need room to be immature and to express the raw, unbridled emotional stirrings that exist inside their hearts. Emotions are neither good nor bad; what matters is how we come to recognize them and to use feeling words to express them responsibly. The goal is to bring a child's emotional world under a system of self-control, intention, decision making, and reflection, but this will not even *begin* to take shape until the 5-to-7 shift (or 7-to-9, for sensitive kids) has occurred. Even then, they will struggle, like adults still do, to temper their reactions in the face of strong emotions. Young children can't get to emotional maturity without a guide—this is one of the ways right relationships were meant to take care of vulnerable hearts and keep them soft.

2. Parents as Shields for Vulnerable, Soft Hearts

The heart is a beautiful symbol to represent the vulnerability that comes with being able to feel one's emotions. The steady hum of the heart beating is like the emotional pulse we take as our child grows. Not only our bodies can get hurt, but our feelings too. If we didn't have feelings, we would never feel scared, lost, sad, or confused, or know the sting of betrayal and disappointment. We would also never feel love, responsibility, fulfillment, hope, or the desire to care and play freely.

Emotions drive growth, and feelings seek consciousness, giving life its vibrancy. They also make us vulnerable to being wounded emotionally. Young children often feel hurt by others; for example, Simon told his mother, "My sister pushed me and hurt my feelings," and "She won't play with me. She is so mean!" Human emotion provides us with a dilemma: we cannot experience euphoric states like love and joy without running the risk of experiencing despair and loss. Love is the doorway through which feelings of loss open up. Feelings of despair come in the wake of losing something we care about deeply.

What is the answer to the paradox presented by human emotion? How can we preserve vulnerable feelings and keep hearts soft in the face of so much heartache? The answer is shields, and there are two possible ones that help filter the world and provide a protective cover for the human heart so that it can stay soft and full of expression: (1) emotional defence mechanisms centred in the brain and (2) right relationships with caring adults.

EMOTIONAL DEFENCE MECHANISMS

What depth psychology has argued for centuries and neuroscientists now support is the existence of emotional defences to protect vulnerable hearts.[7] The brain is equipped to erect defences to inhibit and defend against vulnerable feelings when they are too much to bear and overwhelm the system. Defences are protective mechanisms that allow us to carry on in situations where feelings could keep us from doing what we need to.

Defences are a strategic move by the emotional part of the brain to enable survival in an environment that is too wounding. For example, if a parent continuously yells at or scares a child to get compliance, the constant state of alarm may erect emotional defences so that a child can appear unaffected in the middle of so much emotional turmoil. Under these conditions a parent would have to yell louder to alarm a child and make it over their walls of emotional defence. Emotional defences appear spontaneously and are not under direct conscious control.

Emotional defences need to remain fluid, ebbing and flowing, for development to continue to progress. Developmental problems can arise when the defences get stuck because they decrease the amount of vulnerable feelings that can be felt. When defence mechanisms get stuck, the child no longer experiences the vulnerable feelings they need to for growth to occur, especially the feelings of caring for others and being cared for. Instead of having a soft heart that is moved to tears or exhibits fear when appropriate, they can appear hardened, with little sign of vulnerable emotion.

The vulnerable feelings most likely to be defended against are futility, woundedness, dependence, fulfillment, embarrassment, shame, alarm, caring, and responsibility. Both caring and responsibility are required for the expression of empathy, and if defended against, will be absent in a child's interactions with others. When emotional defences have been erected, a child is less likely to see or hear things that could hurt them. This includes not being able to see one's mistakes, not remembering events that would bring back vulnerable feelings, not being able to see trouble or rejection coming, and significant attention problems. In short, anything that makes you feel bad cannot be seen or heard.

Adults do not typically notice when vulnerable feelings have gone missing in a child. Adults do notice the behaviour problems that arise from the absence of alarm, futility, or caring feelings—for example, a child who doesn't depend on their parent or constantly states, "I don't care" or "It doesn't matter." If these defences are temporary and situational, they will probably pose few problems for the child developmentally. When they are ongoing or necessary because of a wounding environment, they can be costly to the child's overall development. When feelings are numbed on a more chronic level, children's hearts "harden" and vulnerable feelings are absent—which

---

VULNERABLE FEELINGS MORE LIKELY TO BE DEFENDED AGAINST

- feelings of **futility** (sadness, disappointment, grief, sorrow)
- feelings of **dependence** (emptiness, neediness, missing, loneliness, insecurity)
- feelings of **shyness** and timidity
- feelings of **embarrassment** including blushing
- feelings of **shame** (that something is wrong with me)
- feelings of **woundedness** (hurt feelings, anguish, pain)
- feelings of **alarm** (apprehension, unsafe, anxiety, and fear)
- feelings of **caring** (compassion, empathy, devotion, concern, provide for, meet needs of, treasure, invested in)
- feelings of **responsibility** (feel badly, remorse, make things work for, take the lead concerning, make things better for)

Figure 6.4 Taken from Neufeld *Heart Matters: The Science of Emotion* course

affects their potential to mature as social, separate, and adaptive beings.

When four-year-old Annie was separated from her mother because of an extended work project, she was sent to live with her grandmother for three weeks. Annie suddenly stopped being able to see things that would normally alarm her. She played with neighbourhood kids who teased her mercilessly, but she remained unaware of or unaffected by their taunts. Annie also started to have accidents and pee her pants despite being toilet trained. She was even adamant after her wet spots were revealed that it wasn't her who had peed her pants. The vulnerability of being separated from her mother and left with a grandmother she wasn't deeply attached to was too emotionally distressing. Her brain compensated by inhibiting distressing and vulnerable feelings and sensations. This allowed Annie to bear the separation but created a number of other problems. Fortunately, when her mother returned and spent time collecting Annie as well as getting her back into their daily routine, her emotional defences eventually came down and her soft feelings returned. As Annie's emotional system started to thaw, she stopped wetting herself and cried about being left with her grandmother.

The brain can also evoke emotional defences to back out of and avoid attaching to someone because of the anticipation of getting hurt or wounded by them. For example, a father called me frantically after his four-year-old, Aiden, had run away from him at the park after a fight with his brother and cross words from his mother. Aiden had bolted across a busy street without looking and disappeared. When they finally found him, he was hiding in his room. Aiden refused to come out or let anyone near him. As they waited him out and communicated that they were there but wouldn't push him, his emotional defences came down slowly and he reappeared. The parents were alarmed at Aiden's behaviour and sought help in understanding what had happened. When they started to understand Aiden's sensitivity and how easily he was hurt by wounding words, they started using less emotionally provocative ways of dealing with him. Emotional wounding is often the challenge in caring for sensitive children. They can hear the twinge of frustration in a parent's voice or see a frown forming on their face, and their brain can quickly eject them out of the relationship in anticipation of wounding. They may run, hide, not listen or obey, do the opposite of what is expected, and become unmanageable.

For optimal emotional functioning, a child should be able to express a range of vulnerable feelings, such as feeling tired when needing rest, embarrassed when exposed, cautious when alarmed, sorry when bad things happen, hopeful when looking forward, caring about others, or hurt when wounded. Signs that indicate a child's brain may have erected emotional defences include the following:

1. They no longer talk about what distresses them or their hurt feelings.

2. They no longer feel unsafe or alarmed when they should.

3. They no longer see rejections or they can't stay out of harm's way.

4. They no longer adapt to the lacks and losses in their life, which is often accompanied by increased frustration and aggression.

5. They no longer feel emptiness or desire, just a chronic level of boredom.

When a child's brain has moved to defend against being hurt too much, it will fall to the adults in their life to work through their relationship to soften the child's heart.

RIGHT RELATIONSHIPS WITH CARING ADULTS

Right relationships with adults are the ultimate shields for a child's vulnerable heart. Parents are empowered in their shielding function when a child uses them as a compass point to get their emotional bearings. Young children will look to their parents to make sense of what distresses them, preventing the brain from inhibiting vulnerable feelings. A right relationship with a parent gives the child someone to turn to who can take the sting out of shame (when feeling something is wrong with who they are), reduce separation (when being rejected, unwelcome, or uninvited), and lower alarm (when feeling unsafe physically and emotionally). Love is the ultimate shield for a child's vulnerable heart—it is a beautiful design.

Parents and adults need to be the ones to capture a child's heart and hold on to it through their caretaking. If the parent becomes a source of wounding and a child faces too much separation, shame, and alarm, then a child is less likely to turn to them to help with their emotions. Only one adult is required to shield a child's heart, though more are better, to create a larger emotional safety net for a child.

As a shield, a parent can help a child express their feelings in a vulnerable way by coming alongside them. The act of coming alongside involves inviting the child to tell you how they are feeling, reflecting on what you have heard, and acknowledging what it is like to feel this way. When you come alongside their feelings and experiences, you are trying to convey that you understand how they are stirred up and that you are there to help. One of the most important things a parent can do is help bring a child's inner emotional world into their conscious awareness. When you come alongside a child, you are leading them through their emotional experiences.

To come alongside a child's emotions is to refrain from doing the opposite, such as discounting their feelings with statements like "It's no big deal, just go outside and play" or "Don't worry about making mistakes, it is just part of learning." When we overrule or deny their feelings, we fail to create the space they require to recognize, name, and understand their fears, desires, and frustrations. Other unhelpful responses include attempts to rationalize feelings away through logic, such as "Don't let what people say bother you. Their words can't hurt you," or "What do you mean I never buy you anything? Why are you so ungrateful. The other day I bought you..." Our feelings cannot be simply explained away; in fact, we need to look at our jealousy, sadness, and loss in the light of day. Further unhelpful responses to children's emotions include prescriptions for how they should handle something, or seizing the opportunity to teach a lesson: "If you would keep your things more organized, then you would know where to find them when you needed them." Coming alongside a child's feelings should communicate a genuine desire to know what is within a child's heart and to assume responsibility for helping them through their emotional reactions.

For example, a mother said her kindergartner was grumpy about having to go to school and started using the word "stupid" a lot. She got upset with him and told him to stop swearing. When he wouldn't stop, she threatened to take away his time on his iPad for a week, to which he responded by hitting her. She asked me what she should have done and I walked her through what feelings she had missed bringing to the surface that could be achieved by coming alongside her son. She could have said, "I see you are grumpy about having to go to school today," or "It's hard to go to school on Monday after a fun weekend when you get to play and don't have to do work," or "I see you are feeling frustrated this morning. What is going on for you?" Coming alongside her child's frustration would have helped to diminish it, increased his awareness of it, and helped him learn more appropriate words to communicate about it. Young children lack sophistication in understanding their emotional world, and coming alongside helps parents bring vulnerable feelings to consciousness and point the child to how to share them responsibly.

One of the biggest sources of emotional wounding for young children is other children. Young children need strong adult shields to protect their vulnerable hearts from being hardened by wounding peer interaction. Jack was a six-year-old whose parents had come to me for help. Since he was an only child, his parents had arranged regular playdates under the false assumption that he needed peer interaction to learn social skills. As Jack entered kindergarten, he loved spending time with his peers, and by grade 1 he had become peer oriented. He continually asked to be with his peers, was frustrated and bored when away from them, didn't listen to his parents or teacher, and spoke disrespectfully to adults. Once the parents understood the root of the problem as peer orientation, they moved swiftly to reclaim and strengthen their relationship with him. Jack's playdates were cut back, he started having date nights with his parents, they reduced his time in after-school care and on technological devices, they cultivated a stronger relationship between Jack and his teacher, and they brought in his aunties, uncles, grandparents, and younger cousins to foster a natural attachment hierarchy. Within months, they made significant headway and were thrilled when Jack started to listen and turn to them for help.

As Jack drove home with his Dad after school one day, the following conversation unfolded about a bossy boy in his class:

Jack: "Do I have abs, Dad?"

Father: "Abs—what are you talking about?"

Jack: "Caden said I had to lift my shirt to see if I had abs. I did and he said I didn't, and they all laughed."

Father: "Oh, Jack, that must have been hard. How did you feel about it?"

Jack: "I was just really confused because I didn't know what it meant. Caden is always mean to me too. I don't like it."

Father: "I can see how you would feel embarrassed and hurt. Not many people have abs, Jack, and it means they exercise and have a muscular belly. Look at me. Do I have abs? No. See, I have a little bit of flab here. This is okay. You are just like me and most people."

One week later, Jack got in the car after school and said to his dad, "Caden came up to me today and said I don't have abs. I told him no one really does and I'm fine the way I am. Caden just looked at me and didn't know what to say and he just walked away." After Jack's father told me this story he quickly moved on to discuss other matters, but I stopped him and said, "Do you see what you have done for your son?" He looked confused by my question, so I said, "Your son doesn't go to school anymore without the one thing he must always have in his backpack." He still looked unsure, so I said, "You. He never goes to school without you. How you love him just like he is and how he is just like you. It's about keeping strong what you have recaptured." At that point we both stopped because it was so beautiful to see, so clear, and so perfectly laid out before us—he had become the shield for his son's heart.

Research on resiliency over the last 35 years has consistently demonstrated the link between children's emotional health and social success with strong caring relationships with adults.[8] Even when a child is faced with bullying, poverty, addiction, or mental illness in the home, the presence of substitute adults such as grandparents or adults found in schools or churches is the single most protective factor for emotional well-being.[9]

Resilience is one of the most important things we need to cultivate in our children.[10] Unfortunately, the message that relationships are the answer to human vulnerability has not been translated into practice. There is still a movement to teach young children tools, techniques, and strategies to be resilient as if it were something they needed to learn like a school subject. Children were never meant to be responsible for keeping their hearts safe or soft. Resilience arises naturally from right relationships in which adults are the emotional shields in the face of distress. What matters is *who* a child turns to when upset, *who* they tell their secrets to, *who* they shed their tears with, and *who* they trust to guide them. A child needs to resolutely see, feel, and hear the message that a parent believes in them and can be leaned upon. The parent needs to affirm that getting hurt is part of life and that the answer is to hold on to someone who is holding on to you. When children feel they matter to their parents, what other people think of them matters less. We don't need to save our children from the wounding world they live in—this is impossible. It is our job to make sure we don't send them into it empty-handed. At the root of resiliency, emotional vulnerability, and soft hearts lies a simple truth: *whoever* a child gives their heart to has the power to protect it with their own. We need to seize the lead in the attachment dance so that we become the shield our children's soft hearts require.

3. Parents as Tempering Agents

Young children lack internal self-control over their emotions because of immaturity. A mature emotional system will allow them to understand and communicate more responsibly with others, but this requires brain development to get there. The challenge with young children is they experience only one emotion at a time. They are not able to mix and integrate feelings until their brain matures and emotions have been singularly identified. As a result, they have little capacity to temper themselves in the face of their strong emotions. The answer to the emotional impulsivity in a young child is for them to be attached to an adult who has self-control and can act as a tempering agent for the child's emotional energy.

The word *temper* means to serve as a neutralizing or counterbalancing force, to moderate, modify, mitigate, alleviate, reduce, lighten, or soften. It is the perfect word to describe the actions of parents in the face of their young child's strong emotions. Tempering is an active role and doesn't place the responsibility for the emotion on the child's shoulders. Tempering a child's emotions requires reading the child's emotional state and determining the best way to move a child towards emotional stability and balance. The challenge is for the adult not to get lost in their child's emotional response or lose their own temper in the process.

The image that comes to mind when I consider the speed and strength of a young child's emotions is that of a train. When a child is really stirred up, they can take on the energy of a train running down the tracks at breakneck speed. There is little in the way of a braking function to stop them—not to mention the risk of derailment! In the face of such emotional energy, parents feel paralyzed and usually tell the child to stop or cut it out, with little effect. One parent asked in a presentation, "What should I do when my child is hitting and throws things at me?" Her friend sitting beside her replied, "You need to duck and get out of the way." Although we all laughed, the reality is that this action might preserve the parent from getting hit, but it won't instill faith in their caretaking, nor will it protect other vulnerable people from a child's foul frustration. We know emotional energy must be allowed to run in a young child, but how do we assume responsibility for taking care of it?

Parents are meant to take the lead in deciding when, where, how, and who will deal with their child's emotions. This is what a tempering agent does: it reads the child and considers the most effective strategy, under the present conditions, that will allow a child to express, feel, and be restored to emotional balance. When to address a child's emotions could be in the moment or later, when the intensity decreases, or both. Where a child's emotions are addressed can include a private or public space. For example, you could choose to distract them while grocery shopping but invite them to express themselves when you are at home. How you lead a child to their vulnerable feelings could mean talking to them directly, reading a picture book, or helping them express themselves through play. There are many people who can help a child with their feelings, but a parent must decide who has a deep enough relationship to bring the vulnerable feelings to the surface.

Emotional energy must flow; this is nonnegotiable, but the responsibility for creating rest by counterbalancing and neutralizing young children's emotions lies with the parent. For example,

Kai's mother said she had ordered her four-year-old son some model planes, a favourite hobby he shared with his father. As soon as Kai learned about the planes he was excited and began to ask repeatedly when they would arrive. After 48 hours, the mother grew impatient and said, "I've told you the same answer a hundred times—they won't come for another week—stop asking me the same question! Can't you understand you need to wait?" But Kai didn't have the capacity for patience, as this requires the mixing of two feelings— frustration and caring. His desire for his planes was excruciating for him. All Kai was feeling was a strong desire; what was missing were his tears about having to wait for something he wanted right away. His father was the one who responded to Kai's incessant questions by coming alongside his upset and saying, "I know you love these planes and you are so excited to get them in the mail. It is so hard to hear you have to wait. You are so frustrated that they are not here." As his father took this approach, he melted Kai's frustration into tears. As Kai's tears fell, the futility of asking questions about the planes and when they would arrive finally registered and he stopped.

What Kai's story exemplifies is how young children lack the capacity to create order in their emotional system when they are most stirred up. Telling a child to cut something out may reduce or alter expression instead of helping them understand what feelings they are having and what to do with them. This is why parents must become tempering agents and move away from "cut it out" approaches and towards having a neutralizing effect on children's emotional energy.

What our young children would really like us to understand about them is that their emotional immaturity can lead to impulsive, aggressive, inconsiderate, and egocentric behaviour. They need help and guidance in becoming emotionally mature and in being able to relate to others in a responsible way. This means an adult will need to have a relationship with their child's feelings. Parents will need to help their children learn a language of the heart, buy them time until impulse control around emotional content is present, and temper their strong reactions. Children cannot evolve and grow as emotional beings without adult relationships to shield and preserve their soft hearts.

7

Tears and Tantrums
Understanding Frustration and Aggression

Heaven knows we need never be ashamed of our tears,
for they are rain upon the blinding dust of earth, overlying our
hard hearts. I was better after I had cried, than before—more
sorry, more aware of my own ingratitude, more gentle.
CHARLES DICKENS[1]

N THE MIDDLE of a business meeting, Elise's attention was hijacked by a frantic message from her mother-in-law, who was taking care of her three-and-a-half-year-old son, Nathan. In a controlled yet panic-laden voice, Grandma relayed how her grandson was "melting down" on the sidewalk with screams, cries, and refusals to move. When Elise asked what happened, Grandma replied, "I was trying to take him for a sushi lunch like you asked, but he has other plans—he is screaming he wants 'ham-churgers.' I made the mistake of walking by a restaurant that serves them and now he won't listen to me—can you talk to him please?" Elise replied, "All you need to do is say no and comfort him. It's fine if he cries." Her mother-in-law paused long enough for Elise to hear her son wail, "I want fries! I want ham-churgers!" Grandma replied, "He is so loud, he is so upset. I just can't say that. It just breaks my heart to hear him cry and to say no. I can give Nathan the phone so you can tell him no."

As Elise listened to her son cry and to the desperation in Grandma's voice, she knew a sushi lunch was a futile endeavour. She couldn't fix the problem from afar, nor could she risk conveying to Nathan that her mother-in-law couldn't handle him. Elise responded with her best option: "Tell Nathan you've changed your mind and you really want to have hamburgers for lunch too. Tell him you are going to make a Grandma executive decision and take him there." As Elise heard Grandma gasp a sigh of relief, she hoped it would be enough to convince Nathan there was still someone in charge while getting them beyond the impasse.

The force of a young child's frustration can make an adult buckle and run for cover, but this will come at a cost to the adult's capacity to lead a child in accepting limits and restrictions. In the face of tears and tantrums, adults need to know when to change something for a child, know when to help them accept the things they cannot change, and have the wisdom to know the difference.

Toddler Force and Preschooler Hurricanes

YOUNG CHILDREN ARE ferocious and tenacious change agents who strive to get what they want at all costs. Their requests are fuelled by emotion but are disconnected from the constraints of reality. If one cookie was yummy, then a whole bag must be "yummier." Their desires and wishes are untempered by the knowledge that they can't always get what they want, nor do they know what is good for them. They can argue like lawyers, negotiate like salespeople, and demonstrate why whining is the most annoying sound to the human ear, worse than the screech of a high-pitched table saw.[2] This isn't a cruel joke played on parents but a well-designed developmental feature that allows adults to help children adapt to the world they live in. Children are not born with preprogrammed knowledge about limits and restrictions, and for good reason: to allow for flexibility, versatility, and malleability in adapting to their environment. The challenge is, adults must be the ones to present the futilities of life to a child and ride through frustration until they accept those futilities. Failure to do this can foster alpha problems and a lack of resilience when faced with adversity.

Young children can erupt with frustration in their own unique style, including screaming, yelling, kicking, biting, head banging, scratching, pinching, vomiting, or a combination. As one father said, "As soon as my two-year-old son doesn't get what he wants—a chocolate, the chair his sister has, a toy, random items around the house like the dog's tail—he hits, bites, and throws whatever is at hand. He also screams very loudly. There are tears, but these are very angry tears." Ironically, it seems that a child's particular bent for expressing foul frustration can coincide with what is most egregious to their caretaker. Vomit-phobic parents seem to get the pukers, and sound-sensitive parents get the screamers. A mother who adopted a child at birth asked me, "We don't scream or yell in our house. My husband and I are the most peaceful parents, but my daughter has started to throw herself on the ground and scream at the top of her lungs. I am worried—is something wrong with her mental health?" Although I reassured her that tantrums were common in young children, she asked, "But what am I supposed to do when she is like this?"

Parents will attest that early childhood is a violent time because of their young child's lack of impulse control and strong emotions. As Gordon Neufeld states, "It's lucky for us they have small bodies and poor aim."[3] Their frustration can erupt in a second, bringing with it unanticipated challenges and uncivilized behaviour. It can unsettle a parent to see their child lash out, as one mother revealed in a phone message to me: "When my three-year-old punched me in the head today, screaming and kicking as I pulled her out of a store because I said no to buying her something, I realized I need to get some better strategies for dealing with her!" The good news is, a child's untempered reactions should start to dissipate with ideal development, around the time the 5-to-7 shift occurs. Physical forms of aggression should transform into verbal forms, and the child will start to shudder and shake but erupt in aggression less frequently. As one five-year-old said after feeling bad for screaming, "I tried to hold it in, but my neck and mouth couldn't take it any longer."

It is the *mixing of feelings and thoughts* that comes with the 5-to-7 shift that delivers a natural resolution to children's untempered frustration. When a child feels both *frustrated* with someone and also *alarmed* at the thought of hurting that person, the conflict between these feelings will temper their reaction. When they can feel both the *impulse to attack* someone and their *caring not to hurt* someone, they will demonstrate better self-control. The mixing of feelings and thoughts holds their eruptions at a standstill and allows words to become the answer to expressing frustration. With guidance from adults, their words will also transform into more civilized forms of expression—"Poo poo face I hate you, Daddy" will morph into "I'm frustrated. I don't like your answer."

Frustration is often seen as a problematic emotion because it is associated with attacking energy and acts of aggression. However, frustration is not something we need to unlearn; it is an important emotion that is hardwired into humans for good reason. It is a powerful force that has a job to do—frustration is the emotion of change. It is meant to pack a powerful punch, and it isn't something we can run from or extinguish. Frustration is what mobilizes us to work hard at getting what we want or to change the things that don't work for us. We will serve our children well if we can help them harness its power and bring it under a system of intention and decision making by the time they are young adults. They will be able to drive forward and effect change in a way that is civilized and responsible. They will be able to hold themselves and others accountable for what doesn't work and needs to change. We need to help a child understand this powerful reservoir of emotional energy inside of them. Frustration underlies our capacity to change the world around us and ourselves as we mature.

How Do We Help Children with Their Frustration?

FRUSTRATION IS A strong emotion that fuels a young child to change what doesn't work for them. However, they need to be equipped to live in a world where they don't always get what they want. Sometimes they are the ones who need to change, and parents will need to help them let go of their agendas and realize they can survive not getting their way. To do this, adults will need to accept that there is nothing wrong with a young child who has wants and wishes—like eating cookies for breakfast or staying up past bedtime. What is imperative is that adults don't fall short of their responsibility to present life's futilities, which are many, such as helping a three-year-old get to sleep when they claim, "I don't want to go to bed. I'm nocturnal like my hamster."

Helping a child accept something is futile is *not* a logical process but an *emotional* one. They are poor judges of what is futile and need help figuring out which pursuits can be fulfilled and which ones need to be relinquished. They can be incessant in their pursuit of something they want and adults will need to take an active role in helping them rest from futile endeavours. Efforts to talk a young child out of something in a reasonable and rational manner are usually doomed to failure. We need to go through their heart not their head for futility to register. They need to *feel* they are up against the limits and restrictions in life. We need to make it clear to their *heart* that something is not going to happen. We need to help them hear our "no" and be moved to accept it *emotionally*. Just like in a maze, a young child needs to feel where there is a dead end so that they can find another way through. As one four-year-old said when he realized his father wasn't going to change his mind, "Daddy, I don't like your no. I'm telling Mommy on you."

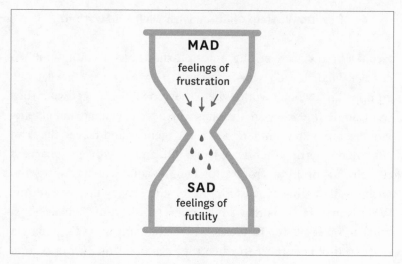

Figure 7.1 Adapted from Neufeld *Making Sense of Aggression* course

A child can accept that something is futile only if they are moved to feel sadness, disappointment, and loss when they cannot effect change. If the child's heart is soft and vulnerable feelings can be felt, mad should eventually move to sad. The feelings of frustration should melt into feelings of futility. It is sad tears (not to be confused with mad tears) that signal an end to their futile pursuit and convey that their brain has got the message that something will not change. The relentless whining, frustration-filled whirring energy of the young child will transform, almost like magic, into sadness or disappointment. Feelings of frustration should come to a standstill and the emotional energy should transform into surrender—the child will be at rest. As a child accepts what cannot change, their eyes might start to water and tears may flow. It is through a path of tears, of feeling sad or disappointed about what cannot change, that young children come to accept the futilities in life and become more resilient and resourceful.

Beatrice was a three-year-old who had fallen in love with candy and asked for it continually, especially for breakfast. After many no's, many sad tears, and much comforting on her mother's part, Beatrice accepted the verdict and stopped asking for it. The mother was taken by surprise one month later when Beatrice asked for candy for breakfast again. A little frustrated, the mother replied with sarcasm, "Sure, you can have as much candy as you want for breakfast. Cookies and cake, too. Don't forget the ice cream in the freezer—get your bowl and fill it up!" Beatrice's eyes widened and her mouth opened, but nothing came out until she gasped and said, "Mama, you would need to be dead for that to happen!" The mother was reassured Beatrice had adapted but her spirit had not been crushed in the process. Beatrice knew candy was off limits for breakfast, but it didn't mean she had to stop desiring it.

The Importance of Tears of Sadness

SAD TEARS OR disappointment are the ways we know futility has registered for a child. As developmental psychologist Aletha Solter states, "When children cry the hurt has already happened. Crying is not the hurt but the process of being unhurt."[4] The capacity to cry tears in the face of emotional distress is uniquely human, according to neuroscientists, supporting Darwin's claim that they are a special form of expression reserved only for us. Tears have been associated with bringing relief, reducing tension, and restoring health. William Frey's research found that tears cried in sadness shed toxic waste products from the blood system.[5] When tears are shed, there is also a release of oxytocin, the attachment chemical that inhibits the biological stress chemical cortisol. When children cry and receive comfort from attachment figures, this also increases oxytocin levels and decreases stress-related ones.[6] In a young child, tears are the best indicator of an emotional system that is functioning well.

One of the problems with tears is that their expression is not equally supported for boys and girls. Current definitions of masculinity pressure parents to suppress boys' tears and vulnerable feelings.[7] Interestingly, this has not always been the case. Tears used to be a sign of virtue and good character in men.[8] When tears are not invited to come forth, they can get stuck, and a child's frustration can move into less vulnerable forms of expression, such as physical aggression.

Despite the restorative effect of tears for both girls and boys, they are threatened in a world that divides emotion into positive and negative categories, where happiness and calm are to be pursued at the expense of sadness and upset. William Blake wrote, "Joy and woe are woven fine,"[9] suggesting that a fulfilling life consists of both happy and sad feelings. When we communicate to our children that there is something wrong with them for being sad, we thwart both their tears and an opportunity to rest from what they cannot change. A lack of support for tears comes at the expense of cultivating adaptation and resilience. Parents sometimes believe tears are a sign they are doing something wrong, whereas they are an indication that a child has trusted them with their heart.

Perhaps the root of societal and cultural resistance to tears is that they convey vulnerability and dependence. Evolutionary biologist Oren Hasson argues that the appearance of tears communicates a lowering of defences to make oneself more amenable to receiving comfort and caretaking.[10] In a world that thrives on independence and pushes young children to grow up too fast, tears are the antithesis to this message. Tears signal dependence and convey a hunger to be cared for. Emotional survival for a young child requires being tethered to a caring adult.

Young children weren't meant to take care of their feelings; they are just starting to learn names for them and don't have control over them. We need to stop shifting our responsibility for a child's upset onto their shoulders with statements such as "Control your temper," "Calm down," "Why can't you figure this out?" "I have told you a hundred times…," "Stop being like that," "Cut it out," "You need to think more positively," and the classic line "Why are you crying?

I'll give you something to cry about." We need to take care of their frustration and tears; they are the clearest signal to us a child needs help. Helping a child understand what is behind their tears is the goal, but children will not share their emotions with just anyone. The ability to help a child cry leads back to the dance of attachment and whether that child depends on a caretaker.

The beautiful thing about tears is they are always seeking expression, just like frustration. Sometimes the doorway to sadness will open in the most peculiar way—a stubbed toe, a broken toy, a lost teddy bear. Some parents are surprised by the volume and intensity of their child's tears once a channel for them opens. When you understand that tears lie waiting to be expressed, it is easier to come alongside seemingly trivial incidents that help them get their tears out. One mother recalled watching her child with autism weep unexpectedly:

> Alex had just emerged out of a year of intense alarm, horrifying phobias, great distress, more than I thought possible for a four-year-old to experience. One day, he was sitting at the computer and found some music, a melancholic madrigal. He was so touched by the beautiful sadness that he started crying. A soft, sad, deep crying—not the screaming, torturous protest I had been hearing all year long. I hadn't heard that kind of crying for so long.

The mother was moved to tears by her son's emotional expression, amazed that this music could have drawn so much out of her son's heart, and truly thankful that it had. One of the best gifts we can give our children is to value their sad tears and make room for them to flow.

A young child is an adaptive being waiting to unfold with the right caretaking by their parents. It is a messy process that is noisy, chaotic, violent, unpredictable, tiring, and rewarding as the fruits of adaptation come to life before our eyes. The best gift we can give a young child is to help them find their sadness and tears when they're up against the things they cannot change. They will be able to learn from their mistakes, be transformed by what they cannot change, and use their frustration to change the things they can. Sometimes the emotional force behind frustration can be quelled only by the surrender our tears bring as we are brought to rest from our futile pursuits. Tears bring a child to rest so that they can play and grow— we must become the tearjerkers and comforters our children require.

Common Childhood Futilities

MAD FEELINGS NEED to transform into sad ones when our children are up against the things they cannot change. Here are fifteen of the most common futilities faced by young children, along with four of the hardest ones for them to deal with.

1. *The futility of trying to hold on to good experiences.* When young children are having a good time, they don't want it to end, and who can blame them? Having to leave Grandma's house or end a play-date or birthday party can provoke frustrated responses from young children. Anytime they have to transition, they have to say goodbye, and this may bring sadness and frustration with it.

2. *The futility of trying to make something work that doesn't.* Young children believe adults can fix whatever doesn't work, from broken toys to bad weather. They may tell us they want sunny weather on a cloudy day, or a store to open when it is closed. Their expectations have little to do with reality and everything to do with their desires.

3. *The futility of trying to possess a parent—or anyone, for that matter.* As soon as a child is born and the umbilical cord is cut, they are never as close to someone again. This doesn't stop them from

trying, and they move to claim and possess people for their own. Sharing their loved one with anyone will be hard and can result in territorial battles.

4. *The futility of wanting to send a sibling back where they came from.* Adapting to a new sibling often involves a path of frustration and many tears about all the things that change, including having less attention, more noise, and shared space. Four-year-old Gabriella said to her pregnant mother, "If you have a girl then I will call her 'Garbage Can' and throw her in the Dumpster. If you have a boy, then I will call him 'Baby' and go and buy him a special present."

5. *The futility of wanting to be smarter than one is.* One of the futilities young children experience when they go to school is how they differ from other kids. They may want to read or throw a ball like another child or become frustrated as they compare their talents. They are not born with the realization that everyone is different and that many things are learned through trial and error. What young children see is the gap between where they are and where they want to be.

6. *The futility of wanting to be perfect or avoid failure.* Young children can become frustrated when they make mistakes or when the images they have in their head don't come to life the way they envisioned. Towers fall to the ground and pictures look better in their imagination, leading to eruptions of frustration. Coming face to face with human imperfection is frustrating and calls for tears.

7. *The futility of trying to control circumstances.* There are many life events we cannot control, such as the passage of time and losing things we love. These can be experienced as very frustrating and alarming to young children. One mother wrote,

I remember my daughter when we first got baby chicks. We had one little one that didn't look very healthy right from the beginning. My daughter named him Humphrey. Over the next three days we rallied for this chick to survive. She cried in anticipation of his death because he was clearly not well. When the chick died, I noticed that a part of me wanted to pretend it didn't happen, to say he's "gone away" or he "died in the night," and remove all evidence of his dead body to avoid her upset. Instead we left him for her to see him dead in the morning. She cried and cried and cried. We buried Humphrey with a little ceremony, and she cried and cried and cried. We talked about Humphrey for months, and still the tears would come. The next time we lost a chicken, about a year later, Jasmine had a few tears, and then said, "The second time is easier."

8. *The futility of trying to turn back time or undo what's been done.* Young children will often change their minds and try to make a different decision retroactively. They will eat their chocolate ice cream only to turn around and tell you they really wanted vanilla. The idea of permanence and not being able to undo what has been done is hard for a young child to grasp and creates frustration.

9. *The futility of trying to make magic work or to defy the laws of nature.* Early childhood is a time when the laws of nature are being learned. A father of a young boy told me his son would erupt in frustration every time he got his ball to a particular place in mid-air, willing it to stay, only to become upset when it dropped to the ground. Seeing the chasm between their imagination and reality can be frustrating.

10. *The futility of wanting to win all the time.* When young children play games, they often want to win—at all costs, even by cheating. They will change the rules to suit their needs or make up new ones along the way. I have heard kids say, "If you win it really

means you're losing, and if you lose it really means you're the winner." One parent was aghast at my suggestion that young children shouldn't always win. She asked, "Are you saying I shouldn't let my five-year-old win at chess each time we play? He's just little." I responded by asking her where she thought it best her child learn about not being the winner all the time. She contemplated this question and conceded that perhaps she did have a role to play in preparing her son for losing on the playground at school.

11. *The futility of wanting to be bigger than one is.* When children compare themselves to others, they may want to be taller, older, or bigger. One five-year-old asked his father, "Can I tell people I am six years old even when I am not?" When his father asked why, he said, "Because everyone in the class is older than me and I want to be six too." The father wisely replied, "You are what you are and you can't change that."

12. *The futility of wanting to be best and first at everything.* Young children have alpha instincts that seek expression, wanting to be first and the best, and to get ahead of other people. "Poor losers" are kids who haven't been helped to accept the futility of expecting to always end up at the top. The jockeying for position among children reveals itself as they butt in front of each other in school lineups. It is important that a young child be prevented from being first all the time and helped to realize that they can survive this too.

13. *The futility of wanting to be wanted where one isn't.* Sometimes young children aren't invited to birthday parties or playdates; sometimes their sibling doesn't want to play with them. Sometimes adults need to help children find their sadness and tears when they face rejection. Often adults hurry to smooth over troubled peer relationships, insisting that all children should be friends, in

an endeavour to avoid hurt feelings. While this is understandable, especially for a child who experiences a lot of peer rejection, it is also important that a young child be able to read where they are not welcomed and respond accordingly.

14.*The futility of wanting to know what's going to happen.* Sometimes young children want to know what is going to happen, often as a result of alarm and feelings of uncertainty, such as on the first day of preschool. Helping a child find their tears about the changes ahead and reassuring them they will be cared for will help ease their alarm and frustration about the unpredictable and the unknown.

15.*The futility of wanting to avoid upset.* Young children often want to avoid upset, such as being sad or bored. They may try to distract themselves or demand stimulation. Part of a parent's role is to help them deal with the upsets that come with life, such as losing a balloon or dealing with ice cream that falls on the ground, and not attempt to prevent them altogether.

The Four Futilities That Are the Hardest to Face

1. *Futility in the face of limits and restrictions.* As soon as a young child starts to walk, their interests and desires come to life as they explore their environment. Children typically don't like limits and restrictions being imposed on them, preferring to do whatever they want. They will insist that they want to play instead of have a nap, go outside without a jacket, or empty cupboards and drawers. Anytime adults place limits and restrictions on a young child, there is bound to be some frustration. It is important to not always use distraction or other measures to avoid upset and to help them find their tears.

2. *The futility of trying to control other people's actions and decisions.* When young children aren't able to control what other people do, they can become frustrated by their inability to alter outcomes. A four-year-old girl told her friend to stop messing up her table as they played house with their teddy bears. He didn't listen, despite her repeated attempts to tell him to stop. In a desperate move she screamed at him and started to jab him with the plastic cutlery. He started to scream, unable to stop her stabbing, and yelled, "It wasn't me. It was my teddy bear." At that point, she started to jab his teddy bear with her fork. It's hard when children realize they can't control what other people do.

3. *Futilities that derive from one's own nature.* Young children often want to master things their body is still learning to do, such as tie their shoes, click in a 5-point harness seatbelt, scale a climbing wall, colour inside the lines, or write their name. Sometimes children have disabilities that make movement or learning challenging. Physical or emotional limitations can be frustrating and call for tears to adapt to what is possible. Sensitive children often need to shed a lot of tears about all the things that do not work for them.

4. *The futility of unachieved fulfillment.* Fulfillment stems from achieving something we desired or wanted, but this isn't always realistic or possible. Sometimes young children don't get what they want, like the pet puppy or kitten they asked Santa for at Christmas. They have desires, agendas, demands, and needs that go unmet, and this will create frustration. As one boy exclaimed, "My brother's birthday is the worst day of my life!" One of the hardest futilities to face based on unmet needs is separation from someone they want to be close to, like a parent who can't be with them. This will raise alarm along with pursuit of their loved one and will be discussed further in chapter 8.

Helping a Young Child Adapt to the Futilities in Life

HOW DO WE help a child when their frustration erupts and spews forth? How do we develop a relationship with their frustration in a way that helps them adapt to the futilities in their life? The Neufeld Frustration Roundabout demonstrates the three possible outcomes to frustration and how parents can help move a child to adapt to what cannot change. Frustration has three possible outcomes when it is stirred up: (1) the child tries to *change* what does not work for them, (2) the child *adapts* to what they cannot change, or (3) the child moves to *attack*.

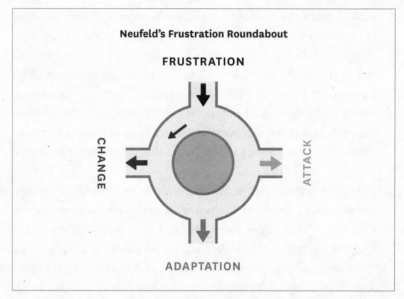

Figure 7.2 Taken from Neufeld *Making Sense of Aggression* course

1. **A Child Moves to Change What Does Not Work for Them**

   When a child is frustrated, one of the first things they may try to do is effect change by begging, pleading, or whining. Their frustration will disappear if a parent concedes to their request, but this is a judgement call that a parent makes each time. Considerations include the timing, the setting, and who will be saying no and dealing with the potential upset. A parent shouldn't say no just to prove a point. A child's capacity to adapt will be taxed when they are exhausted, hungry, or sick, making their frustration overwhelm them more easily.

If a child can't accept a "no" in a particular area, such as candy for breakfast, then the parent may want to represent futility on this issue until the child has accepted the limits and restrictions. If a parent always concedes, distracts, or bribes a child to avoid upset and tears, a child will have few experiences to adapt to and this will negatively impact their overall resiliency. If a child sees that a parent is continuously fearful or unsure how to handle their frustration, alpha problems can also arise. It is important that a parent read the child and the situation to determine when to say no and when to fulfill the child's desires.

If a parent isn't willing to meet a child's request, the child's frustration may be directed at changing the parent's mind, starting with questions such as "Why can't I?" A young child can be a relentless change agent who refuses to take no for an answer. The fatal mistake is telling them *why* you are saying "no" at this point. Parents can end up trapped in a logical conversation with their young child, with arguments made and countered, negotiations sought and refused. In the face of a child's incessant whys, parents can simply reflect that it is frustrating not to get the answer they want.

Two parents came to see me about the continuous debates they were having with their young child every time they said no, which led to extended tantrums. Upon closer examination, it became clear they were getting caught in a logical, circular conversation.

Teddy: "Please can I have another cookie, Daddy? They are so yummy."

Father: "No, you just had one now and earlier today too. "

Teddy: "But you said I could have one after dinner."

Father: "I did give you one after dinner. That is it."

Teddy: "But why can't I have more? They are too little."

Father: "Because I said so. Cookies aren't good for you."

Teddy: "I ate all my vegetables. Please can I have one?"

Father: "No more cookies. I told you they're not good to eat before you go to bed."

Teddy: "Mommy lets me have more cookies. I want one more."

I asked the parents if they could just say no in a firm but caring way and avoid arguing and explaining their reasons to Teddy. He wasn't able to hear their "no" because when they argued with him, he thought he still had a chance to change their minds. Both parents began to laugh at my suggestion and said, "Deb, we are both lawyers, this is what we do all day—we argue, we debate, we are logical. It's so hard coming home to a preschooler. They require a totally different skill set." I wholeheartedly agreed and encouraged them to say no without negotiating so that they would help Teddy realize when things were futile.

2. A Child Adapts to What They Cannot Change

If we want a child to adapt to something that is futile, then we need to close the doorway to change and open the doorway to adaptation. Closing the doorway to change means we provide a clear and direct "no" to their request or agenda with little explanation. If the answer sinks in and futility registers emotionally, a child can be moved to adapt, can feel disappointment or sadness, and might even begin to cry. Sad tears signal that the doorway to adaptation has opened and a child is being changed by what they cannot have. In the wake of these tears, resilience and resourcefulness will arise. Once the child has accepted the parent's answer and adapted, then it is fine to share the reasons for the "no," as they are no longer moved to argue against those reasons.

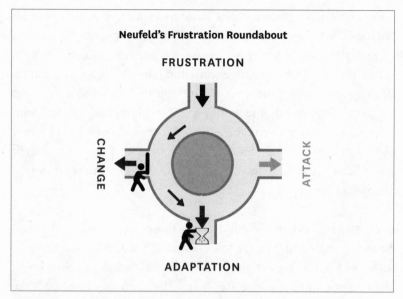

Neufeld's Frustration Roundabout

Figure 7.3 Taken from Neufeld *Making Sense of Aggression* course

When a child is frustrated and cannot effect change, the goal is to move them from "mad to sad." For this to happen, a child must be capable of having sad tears and have a good relationship with a caring adult who will help them get there. The adult needs to hold a young child in their frustration until the doorway to adaptation opens up. This is more of an art than a science and involves a three-step dance manoeuvre in which the parent becomes a double agent of both futility and comfort.

STEP ONE To present what is futile, a parent needs to be clear about what cannot change. For example, "No, we are not taking your sister back and her name will not be Garbage Can."

STEP TWO Holding a child in the experience of frustration means drawing out the frustration and coming alongside it, instead of arguing against it, discounting it, or punishing a child for it. For example,

"I know it's hard to have a new baby sister. You want things to go back to how they used to be." The child may reply with, "Yes! I don't like my sister—take her away!" Again, it is about holding the child in the futility of trying to change something that isn't going to change: "No, we are keeping your sister. I know you are frustrated with all the changes." Importantly, the parent is not trying to talk the child into liking their sister or to convince them they need to be a good brother or help out with the new baby. It isn't about talking them out of their frustration but about dancing them into sadness about what cannot change.

STEP THREE   When the child seems more receptive and the futility is starting to sink in, try to draw out the sadness some more: "I know you're feeling sad about the changes. You liked it just being the two of us, and now we are three." The child may lament, "Take her back, oh, please. I don't want to be a big sister," as the tears start to fall. A parent should ideally be able to read the signs when their child's frustration is softening and they are moving towards surrender. Whatever it takes to get the child over this hump is what a parent should aim to provide—a hug, a touch, silence, patience, or words such as "I am here and this is hard."

The dance from mad to sad is different with every child, as their emotions vary in intensity and vulnerability. A parent needs to read the cues, trust that mad will shift to sad, and hold course through the storm. A mother of a four-year-old relayed the following story in a parenting class one evening about the challenges in riding the frustration roundabout:

THREE-STEP DANCE OF ADAPTATION

· **STEP ONE:** Present the Futility
· **STEP TWO:** Hold in the Experience
· **STEP THREE:** Draw out the Sadness

Figure 7.4 Taken from Neufeld *Making Sense of Aggression* course

It all started when Chloe pushed her brother off a chair and insisted that it was hers. Ben started to cry, so I picked him up and told Chloe she couldn't have the chair. She launched into a tantrum and threw herself on the floor, screaming, "I want that chair!" I just let her scream, but my husband was nearby and asked, "What are you doing? You can't let her do that." I told him, "She's frustrated and she needs to get it out." I told Chloe I was here to give her a hug and understood it was frustrating. My husband whispered to me, "You're going to give her a hug for that?"

It was hard, but I stuck out the crying, the wailing, the stomping, the hand thumping on the floor until I heard the sound that lets me know we are near the end—"Mama, Mama, I want to go home." It's like I can hear the gears shifting downwards inside her head, the sad tears start to fall, and I can finally move in to hug her. In my head all I can think is, "Sweet surrender at last—thank goodness!" and then I realize how tired I am.

I get that it's hard for my husband to understand what to do when she is so upset; he is still learning to feel his way through her tantrums. When she is upset like this, I just long for the tears to come, and do my best to hold on to her frustration and not to make matters worse.

The parents in the group acknowledged how tiring a child's frustration can be to deal with as well as the need for emotional self-control. The mother added that although she isn't always as patient as she would like to be, she was surprised at how good it felt knowing that she could help her child find her tears.

To open the door to adaptation, a child needs a safe place to cry and a safe person to cry with. There are many reasons why adults struggle with helping a young child find their tears, the most common being lack of awareness of what is needed, lack of cultural support for and wisdom regarding intense emotions, fear of upset or of the child's reactions, a compulsive need to make things work for a child, overdependence on reason, and lack of a strong enough relationship to bring the child to tears. When young children are frustrated and up against what they cannot change, they need agents of comfort who will hold on until their frustration can be released through their sadness or disappointment.

It is important to note that if a child does not have a soft heart or cannot shed tears in a vulnerable way, holding them in frustration will lead to escalating attacking energy. The first order of business will be to restore the child's emotional vulnerability, as discussed in chapters 4, 5, and 6, before proceeding with helping them adapt to futilities in their life. Furthermore, a parent can't present something as being futile unless they can control the circumstances around it. Areas such as toilet training, eating, sleeping, or any hygiene chores require the child's cooperation, so holding them in futility here is hard. Battles around these types of activities are addressed in chapter 9. Most importantly, a parent doesn't have to say no to every futility a child is up against and may choose to make something work for them too.

3. The Child Moves to Attack

When a child cannot feel the futility of changing something and the tears do not come, they will be moved to attack. There are many forms of attack depending on the sophistication of the child, including hitting, biting, throwing, tantrums, screaming, shaming, insults, sarcasm, put-downs, and even, for sensitive children, self-attack. Adults often intervene by asking an attacking child why they are so angry—"Why did you throw the toy?" or "Why did you hit your brother?"—which is a request for logic and reason. A child is moved to attack by the emotion of frustration; this is where a parent needs to focus. One mother described how she got caught up in her child's attacking behaviour and missed how frustrated her son really was:

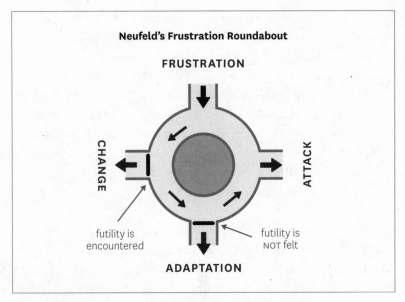

Figure 7.5 Taken from Neufeld *Making Sense of Aggression* course

When my son was about 3 he started randomly scratching kids in the face. It was infrequent, but we were alarmed at the behaviour and very confused about where it was coming from. I tried the usual "This is inappropriate," cut-it-out approach, to no avail. I was embarrassed, frustrated, and couldn't make sense of it. Looking back, I see there were many things frustrating him, and that was his outlet when it got too much.

The challenge with aggression is that when we focus on a child's attacking behaviour, we lose our intuition about the frustration that is driving it. This often leads to the use of consequences and isolation to make a child cut it out and stop. These types of disciplinary tactics will only increase a child's frustration. A mother of a five-year-old relayed the following story of how a well-intended response backfired and exacerbated her daughter's attacking behaviour:

Alice asked for some stickers in a store and I said no. She had a meltdown. An older lady saw us and came over intending to help. She started talking to Alice and told her if she wasn't quiet, Santa Claus wouldn't bring her any presents. Alice let out a ferocious roar. What possessed this woman to use a threat to deal with my daughter's frustration?! Couldn't she see she was only adding fuel to the fire? Now Alice believed she wasn't getting stickers AND Christmas presents! I was so frustrated, I almost had a tantrum on the lady. Instead I told Alice Santa always comes to our house and it was okay that she was frustrated.

When a young child is full of attacking energy, the goal is to direct them back around the frustration roundabout to the door of adaptation by allowing some attacking energy to be vented, coming alongside their frustration, and making it safe for them and others. The goal is to lead them back to their sadness or tears. If a child has lost their tears and there is little sign of vulnerable feelings such as caring and sadness, then the goal will be to survive the incident with everyone's dignity intact. For example, a parent might say, "This isn't working. We are going to do something different," or "I can see you are frustrated. We will talk about this later." When tears are stuck, the focus *must* go to restoring the emotional system before proceeding towards adaptation.

If a parent responds with frustration to their child's attacking behaviour, this will increase the child's aggression and close the door to adaptation. A young child's attacking energy is provocative for parents and often brings forth emotional responses from them. One parent described a time she could have responded differently to her daughter's frustration:

We bought my four- and two-year-olds an expensive kitchen for Christmas. Money is tight for us, but we thought this was something they would really enjoy. One moment, they were looking at it, enjoying it, touching it, and exploring it. The next moment, my oldest had a very frustrated expression on her face and pushed over the kitchen. I was sooo frustrated. I interpreted this as ungratefulness. My daughter tried to open a door or drawer and it didn't work. She was very frustrated and pushed it over. She was not "ungrateful" but very frustrated. I am sorry to say I didn't do a good job dealing with her frustration and aggression, nor did I have a gracious invitation for all of her feelings. And I'm guessing that this is the struggle of many parents—to find their own mixed feelings so they can invite all that is within their children, even if it is foul frustration.

When a child is full of attacking energy, there are three relational principles to bear in mind so as to preserve one's relationship with a child:

1. *Depersonalize the attack.* If the child is kicking, screaming, or biting, telling the child they are mean, bad, disappointing, and so forth will only increase their frustration and attacking energy. Depersonalizing the attack makes it about their behaviour but doesn't convey judgement about it—for example, "Legs aren't for kicking" or "Teeth aren't for biting people."

2. *Focus on the frustration to preserve dignity and come alongside.* Coming alongside a child's feelings can help neutralize their frustration and bring them back around the roundabout to adaptation. For example, a parent might say, "Your teeth have bites in them because you are frustrated. I am going to help you with this." It is important to preserve the child's dignity when they are erupting so as to avoid adding to their frustration and alarm.

3. *Convey that the relationship can take the weight of their emotions.* When a child is attacking, the biggest threat they experience is a loss of

contact and closeness with their parent. When a parent conveys what doesn't work, they need to convey that the relationship is still intact. This may mean telling the child, "I know you are having a hard time. I am still here," or "We're okay. I know you are upset. We'll get through this." The parent needs to take responsibility for preserving the relationship and not hold contact and closeness for ransom until the child apologizes. When separation is used in the face of a child's attack, it will exacerbate the frustration and increase the likelihood of attack.

Frustration and Tears in Sensitive Children

FOR SENSITIVE CHILDREN, tantrums can be more intense, prolonged, and challenging in terms of getting them to tears. Their strong desires and caring can set them up for tremendous disappointment. They often imagine far more than they can ever actualize and become easily frustrated by their human imperfections. Their feelings can be big, overwhelming, and out of control. They need strong caretakers who can help them move through these storms, providing rest and reprieve from a world that feels too much. The challenge is that sensitive children often feel that they are too much for their parents to handle, are too big in their responses, and easily overwhelm others. It is critical that caretakers respond in ways that convey that they can take care of them and handle their behaviour and emotions, as well as ensure that separation is not used as a consequence or punishment.

There are three things that are helpful to consider when managing a sensitive child's frustration and tears:

1. *Protect them from experiences that are too much.* When environments, relationships, and experiences are too much for a sensitive child, their caretakers need to read the situation and protect them accordingly. For example, a parent may sign a young child up for

a music class only to experience them running for the door each time the noise starts. The child may find visual or auditory stimuli overwhelming, and as a result need to spend shorter times in these environments, if any. Pushing them beyond their limits typically leads to the sensitive child either shutting down or exploding with upset. However, it is important for the adult to read what a child is capable of, even in small doses, and not shelter them altogether.

2. *Lead them into vulnerable territory.* Sensitive children are known for their avoidance of upsetting and alarming experiences. They may shy away from sad stories in books and get scared watching children's TV shows. Parents need to walk them gently in these directions when needed and invite them to express what they are experiencing instead of pushing them forward. The sensitive child may try to deflect attention from their feelings, so reading the cues as to what is most difficult helps the adult understand what stirs them up most. When upsets happen, they may need a cooling off period to reduce the intensity of the experience. Afterward, they will be better able to talk about what stirred them up, but they will probably require an adult to lead them there. Acknowledging their feelings, naming and normalizing them, helps them form a better relationship with their internal world that often feels too overwhelming and busy.

3. *Debrief overwhelming situations outside the incident.* When discussing problem behaviour, it is best to deal with it outside the incident, in the context of a warm relationship, and touch the issue gently. Incidents are best deferred to when intense feelings have subsided. In the heat of the moment a parent can simply inform a child, "The behaviour isn't okay and we will talk about it later." A child may reply, "I don't want to talk about it," to which a parent should respond that they will make it easy, quick, and as pain-free

as possible but that sometimes things need to be said and dealt with. When conveying what didn't work, a parent needs to make sure to communicate that the relationship is still okay.

Alarmed by Disconnection
Bedtime, Separation, and Anxiety

---

*And Max the king of all wild things was lonely and wanted to be where
someone loved him best of all.*

MAURICE SENDAK[1]

"I DON'T LIKE TO sleep," yelled four-year-old Sadie midway into her bedtime routine. "It's not fair—you get to sleep with each other and I have no one!" Emily and Dan had grown weary of bedtime battles with Sadie and felt they were being held hostage each night. They were working hard to follow a bedtime ritual and be patient, but getting Sadie to sleep had become a nightmare.

When I asked them to describe how the battles unfolded, Emily said she usually worked from home in the evening, leaving Dan to do the bedtime routine. Sadie enjoyed being told stories and cuddling but not being left on her own. One night, all was going well until Dan went to leave her room, when Sadie jumped up in her bed and demanded that he stay. Dan told her, "It's time for bed and you need to go to sleep. You're going to be tired tomorrow if you don't." Sadie pleaded with him, "No, Daddy, please stay! I don't like the dark!" Dan turned on her night light and said, "You have to go to sleep. I have some work to do and so does Mommy." Dan settled Sadie back into bed and promised to check on her. He was gone five minutes when he heard Sadie run down the hallway in search of her mother to ask for some water. Seeing her, he said, "I told you I would check on you. Now back to bed, Sadie, it's time to sleep. You can't keep doing this. You need to calm your body down and get to bed." With great protest Sadie was led back to bed, where she said, "Daddy, please don't go. I want you! Where's Mommy? I want Mommy!" Dan said he was so frustrated he told her to stay in her bed and walked out of the room. Sadie started to cry but seemed to settle down, until Dan heard a crash coming from her room. He ran to see what had happened and saw Sadie lying on the floor. He rushed to pick her up and said, "Sadie, are you okay? What happened? Why are you on the floor?" She replied, "Oh, Daddy, my stuffed animals threw me out of bed!" Exasperated, Dan put Sadie back to bed but had a hard time calming her down.

Emily and Dan were desperate. They asked, "What's wrong with her? What are we supposed to do? We are so tired and frustrated." I replied, "Young children don't do separation. Separation is alarming for them. When you leave Sadie's room, all she feels is your absence. Bedtime represents up to a 10-hour stretch when you seem unreachable to her because she is unconscious. No one is waiting to be with her in her dreams. She is all by herself, and this is what alarms her. The bedtime routine is like a reflection for the attachment dance you have with a child. How you separate from them is as important as how you invite them to attach to you—separation and attachment are intertwined as far as human connection is concerned." Dan and Emily thought about it and asked, "Well, how do we change it, then?" I replied, "You need to help her rest at bedtime by turning her face into connection instead of separation."

Young Children Weren't Built for Separation

ATTACHMENT IS THE doorway through which separation opens up; attachment and separation are like opposite sides of the same coin. Human connection is our greatest need; therefore, real or anticipated separation is the most powerful of all experiences. Bedtime, good-byes, and transitions represent a departure of some kind, and this is why young children struggle with them. Young children face disconnection from the moment the umbilical cord is cut. We need to grow them into independent, social, and separate beings who can go to sleep, play on their own, attend school, and eventually leave home. The answer lies not in teaching them how to separate but in making it easy for them to separate. They will let go of us when they feel we are holding on to them. In other words, if separation is the problem, attachment is the solution.

Disconnection is provocative for young children because their capacity for relationship is not fully developed. It takes six years of strong development to realize the capacity for deep relationships as discussed in chapter 4. Young children are still developing a sense of self, which makes them highly dependent on the adults around them. The more immature and dependent a child is, the more difficult separation will be. We shouldn't hold their desire for contact and closeness against them but be grateful that they desire contact and closeness with us. If a young child can't be with us, we need to make sure they have a substitute adult who will cultivate a strong connection with them. At bedtime, we need to draw their attention to the anticipation of being with us in order to reduce the separation they face.

What Is Separation Alarm?

FEAR IS ONE of the oldest human emotions, and for good reason. According to neuroscientist Joseph LeDoux, the brain is a sophisticated alarm system that is activated by fear to move us to caution.[2] As an alarm system, the brain is vigilant and highly attuned to threats. Attachment is our most preeminent need; therefore, separation is perceived as the greatest threat and can activate a strong alarm response.[3] Young children, like the young in all other mammal species, possess a separation cry that is meant to draw their caretakers near.[4] This alarm response isn't a mistake or a problem but part of a sophisticated system that is meant to tether adult and child together. A young child's emotional system will be preoccupied with whether someone is taking care of them. When they face separation, their clinging, clutching, restless, frantic, vocal, and possessive actions are all forms of pursuit meant to reduce the distance between them and their attachment figures. If no one consistently comes to their aid, this can activate emotional defences to numb and tune out the distress.[5]

Facing separation can be overwhelming for young children, and it doesn't matter if the separation is real or anticipated. As soon as a child realizes they have to go to daycare, to bed, or to the other parent's house, they may erupt in alarm or frustration over the anticipated disconnection. The experience of separation is dependent on how a child is attaching and is subjective in nature. As discussed in chapter 4, a child attaches in sequence by the senses, sameness, belonging and loyalty, significance, love, and being known. Separation alarm is rooted in the loss of contact and closeness in one of these six ways of attaching.

Separation alarm comes when there is a threat of not being with someone, not being like them, not belonging, not mattering, not being loved, or not being known. For example, one mother told me how her daughter became alarmed when she couldn't hold on to her through her *senses*:

> My daughter can become deeply anxious at night and wants to hold on to me physically. She needs to hear us in the house or see us. One day, after she had fallen asleep, I was sitting downstairs reading. She woke up and came to find me in high alarm. Because I was reading, the house was too quiet and she thought I had left the house and her. I now always read upstairs or with the TV or radio on for background noise.

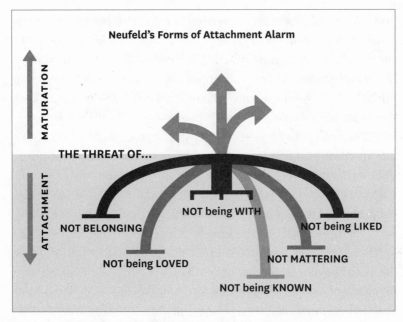

Figure 8.1 Taken from Neufeld *Making Sense of Anxiety* course

An aunt visiting her two-year-old nephew was trying to connect with him through *sameness* and noticed his alarm when she pointed out their differences:

> He was slow to warm up to me, but as I started to read to him, I said, "We're so much alike; we both love to read books." He asked for another book, and when he chose it I said, "That's one of my favourites." He was beaming at me and asked what else I liked. At one point he said, "Do you like marshmallows?" I forgot in the moment about the "sameness" form of attaching and said, "Not so much." The disappointment and alarm on his face broke my heart, and I immediately went back to talking about all the ways we are alike, which brought the smiles back.

Young children are routinely afraid of the dark, being left behind, or being forgotten. All of these themes represent separation from the people they are most attached to. Four-year-old Maggie started to cry and scream for her mother one night five minutes after being put to bed. She wept and said, "Mama, I had a bad dream. The roof got ripped off and I got sucked up to Jupiter and you couldn't come to get me." The answer to Maggie's fear of space travel is not a logical one but an emotional one that addresses her separation alarm. Luckily, her mother didn't argue with her about intragalactic travel but said, "I always know where you are and will take care of you." What young children need to hear over and over again is that an adult is holding on to them—especially at bedtime, the biggest disconnect of the day.

There are many potential sources of separation in a young child's life, such as a new sibling, parents' jobs, school, house moves, daycare, divorce, and adoption. There are also hidden sources of separation, such as becoming their own person and growing more independent. As children evolve into separate beings, alarm is created in the wake of moving away from their parent's caretaking and being able to "do it myself!" The answer for parents, to reduce separation alarm, is to continually work on deepening their attachment and inviting a child to depend on them.

Young children face separation in many ways that can alarm them, such as not being wanted or chosen, or not being the favourite or understood. When they face these alarming futile desires, they may need help finding their tears and being brought to rest. One of the hardest futilities to face is the passage of time and the inevitability of death. Young children may not want to be older on their birthday, may be upset when they lose a tooth, or may tell you they want to stay little forever as if to forgo the passage of time. They can also become aware of existential issues and the finite nature of life through the loss of a pet or an extended family member. These events point their faces into the ultimate separation and can lead to questions such as "Are you going to die too?" Sensitive children can quickly catch on to the possibility of separation and can be quite stirred up as a result. A parent of a sensitive four-year-old noticed her daughter was more alarmed following her birthday and after hearing about her neighbour's dog dying:

> I was checking in on Matilda after putting her to bed when I noticed these bumps where her feet were. I lifted the blanket and saw she was wearing her new black shiny shoes. I asked her why and she started to cry, "Oh, Mama, I just love my shoes. I don't want my feet to grow bigger. Will you buy me another pair when they do?" I told her yes and then said that she would never get too big that I couldn't take care of her. Matilda became very quiet and then asked me, "Mama, when you are dead, will you still love me from heaven?" I managed to tell her, "Yes, I will always be with you. There will never be a day when you will be separated from my love."

The way we help our children face some of the most alarming futilities of life, such as the passage of time and death, is to point their faces into attachment. We can assure them that we will always be their parent, we will always love them, and we are only a thought or a feeling away. When a child loses someone they love, we can help them hold on to this person through stories, pictures, and possessions.

One of the best ways to help a young child make sense of the alarming separations in life is to present them in a non-alarming way. For example, nature, plants, animals, seasons, and the cycle of the moon and the sun all represent the passage of time or the rhythmic flow of life. The best preparation for the separations that lie ahead, such as losing a grandparent, is through natural representations of life and death. Pets are an obvious place to help children understand the futilities that are part of life. One mother said, "I got a fish tank with a lot of guppies in it, but they seemed to keep dying on me. My kids were so upset every time a fish died, I even found my

184 REST, PLAY, GROW

four-year-old kneeling on the floor and praying to the fish in heaven. I used to tell them I must be buying all the really, really old fish and this was the reason they were dying."

If we have to introduce things that could alarm a young child or that suggest we can't keep them safe, like performing earthquake drills or practising emergency lockdowns in schools, the best way forward is through a non-alarming approach. Give them simple instructions, just like a flight attendant does, by conveying essential safety information in a matter-of-fact, friendly way. We don't want to add more alarm by pointing their faces into too much separation; they are far too immature for some of life's most alarming separations. The challenge with young children is that their attachment needs are high, immaturity renders them dependent, and they live in a world that is full of separation.

Anxiety in Young Children

ANXIETY AND FEAR-BASED disorders are the most common mental health problems among children today.[6] Signs of elevated alarm can include excessive tantrums, avoidance of certain situations or stimuli, nausea, stomach or headaches, and refusal to sleep on their own, go to preschool or daycare, or even speak.[7] Children with anxiety may have frequent nightmares, be full of fear and/or be fearless, and have phobias and obsessions, scattered attention, muscle spasms or nervous tics, restless energy, agitation, or a heightened startle response. They may also engage in compulsive anxiety-reducing behaviours such as sucking, chewing, biting nails, twirling hair, rubbing genitals, eating, or continuously seeking comfort from a transitional object like a teddy bear.

When young children are highly alarmed, it can be confusing for adults to determine what separation the child is facing that is stirring them up. When something is alarming and distressing for too long, the brain's emotional defences can move to inhibit vulnerable feelings and perceptions. For example, a child may no longer talk about the bully who bothers them at daycare or school and may even start to play with that person despite being treated poorly. The child will still be alarmed but will no longer be sure why. The real source of their alarm may be blocked from conscious awareness to allow the child to function in an alarming situation or setting. When the brain's emotional defences protect the child from seeing the true cause of their alarm, they may tell you they are scared but will be unable to tell you the cause of it or will make up a reason. In short, anxiety is being alarmed but also blind to its true source. The goal is not to change the child's thoughts or feelings about being afraid but to consider the source(s) of separation and work to change the child's environment or draw out tears where needed. Young children should not be responsible for making themselves feel safe or keeping their hearts soft. This is the role of their caregivers.

There are many sources of separation that underlie the escalating anxiety levels and heightened alarm in young children today. Some of the most common include chronic anticipation of separation and the use of separation-based discipline. Peer-oriented and alpha children can also display high levels of anxiety, as discussed in chapters 4 and 5.

1. Chronic Anticipation of Separation

Young children face unprecedented levels of separation from the people they are attached to, not only because their parents may work outside the home but because of increased divorce rates, geographic mobility, and lack of access to extended family. They are also more likely to be placed in early learning programs and structured activities, which can take them away from their closest attachments at an age when their relational needs are the highest.[8]

When considering whether a child is facing chronic levels of separation, the questions to ask are:

1. How much overall separation does a child face from their closest attachments?

2. Who takes care of a child, is the child attached to them, and, if so, how?

3. Is the child receiving consistent caretaking that provides a generous invitation to attach to their adult(s)?

4. What is the child's developmental capacity to hold on to a parent when apart? and

5. How sensitive is the child, and how provocative is separation for them?

A five-year-old who is attaching to their parents through love is capable of greater separation than is a newborn who is attaching via the senses. The newborn will need consistent care and a generous caretaker who is invested in developing a deep attachment. How does a parent do this in the context of their life? Or can they share this with a substitute caretaker who can provide the same thing?

What is undeniable is every family faces their own challenges and that families have different levels of support and resources, and therefore different choices when it comes to child care, employment, and living arrangements. Many parents need to share the task of raising their child with other adults. Parents will need to cultivate attachment villages to raise their children in, which is addressed later in discussions on using *bridging and matchmaking* to deal with separation alarm.

2. The Use of Separation-Based Discipline

The use of separation-based discipline, such as time-outs, withholding of what a child cares about, or emotional disconnection from an adult, erodes attachment and can lead to increased separation alarm in a child. If a child anticipates that they will be separated because of their behaviour, it can lead to insecurity, as they can't take for granted that their need for contact and closeness will be met. Parents often feign separation on playgrounds when their child is uncooperative or resistant to leaving. They may tell the child, "Goodbye, then. I'm going to leave you at the park if you don't come with me now," which activates the child's separation alarm and can send them running towards the parent. The continued use of separation-based discipline can overwork the child's alarm system and erect emotional defences to numb out the distress.

Alicia and Stephen consulted me about their five-year-old son, who was having regular tantrums at home and at school, wasn't sleeping well, was continually restless, and had trouble paying attention. Seth broke all the rules in his kindergarten classroom and was sent to the principal's office routinely but told his teacher, "I don't care." The teacher was trying to use a sticker reward chart to get him to behave, but he didn't care about her or her stickers. In considering the sources of separation in Seth's life, it was clear that discipline was a major source, with the prevalent use of time-outs and emotional withdrawal and the overuse of consequences. Seth had lost many things he was attached to, from his bike to soccer, his favourite activity. The frequent use of separation-based discipline had eroded his relationship with his parents and resulted in escalating alarm and frustration problems. The more alarm and frustration he expressed, the more discipline he received, fuelling his separation problem.

When Seth's parents stopped using separation-based discipline, started collecting him, and made room for more emotional expression, he began to cry many tears. The tears didn't stop for some time, and his pursuit of his parents increased while his resistance to their directions decreased. When Seth was told he would never be put in a time-out or have his favourite things taken away again as punishment, he immediately went and got sticky notes. On each note he wrote his name, and he started placing them on his favourite objects around the house. His brain had received the message that it was safe enough to connect to things again as well as to people. It took time and patience to reestablish a relationship with Seth, but as his parents did, he started to rest in their care, play on his own, and listen to his teacher, and he was less agitated. Alternatives to separation-based discipline are discussed in chapter 10.

How to Use Attachment to Deal with Separation Alarm

THE ANSWER TO too much separation is to point the child's face into its antidote—attachment. We need to communicate that we are holding on to them so that they can rest in our care. We can do this in a number of ways: by (1) reducing separation, (2) bridging the distance, (3) matchmaking, and (4) reducing their alarm through tears and cultivating resilience.

1. Reducing Separation

When a child is facing too much separation, it is important to look for ways to reduce it both physically and psychologically. A parent may be able to decrease time spent in daycare, preschool, or kindergarten if warranted. They may also trim away non-essential activities that do not foster a relationship with their child or that even interfere with cultivating one, such as structured events and playdates. The parent can look for ways to invite dependence by helping a child get dressed, sharing a hobby with them, or going on outings. Exchanging separation-based discipline practices for more attachment-safe and developmentally friendly ones will also be imperative. If there is undeveloped attachment with a significant adult in their life, for example, a five-year-old who is attaching through sameness (appropriate at age 1 to 2), then deepening this relationship will help reduce the separation. When a child is alarmed, an adult will need to make some room for their feelings and take care of them, such as by staying with them until they fall asleep or keeping them close when they're at home together. Whoever is responsible for the child will need to take a strong alpha stance by reading the child's needs and taking the lead in meeting them.

2. Bridging the Distance

Bridging is an attachment ritual that points a child's face into connection. Instead of focusing on the separation, the child is encouraged to hang on to something that represents attachment with the people who are closest to them. When we create a bridge, we are helping the child focus on what stays the same and connects us despite the divide that has opened up between us. Bridging can be done whenever separation opens up, whether that involves going to bed, attending school, going between two homes, or addressing problem behaviour. Bridging will work to reduce separation alarm only when the child has a right relationship with their adult. If the alarm is caused by peer orientation or alpha problems, getting the child back into right relationship is the first order of business.

Bridging involves giving the child something tangible to hold during their separation as well as focusing on the next point of connection. For example, one mother gave her four-year-old son a picture of her in a plastic bag and put it in his back pocket. She told him she was in his pocket if he missed her at preschool. He came home one day and said, "Mommy, I missed you so much today, I just pulled you out of my pocket and kissed your face." Another mother gave her daughter a locket with their family picture in it. She told her daughter, "If you ever miss us there are neverending kisses and hugs in your locket to use." The mother measured how much missing her daughter experienced each day by asking how many kisses and hugs she needed.

Sometimes daycares and preschools will hang family pictures around their classroom so that loved ones are only a glance away. Notes in lunch boxes are a form of bridging. As you leave a child, you can help reduce separation alarm by focusing on the reunion and what you will do together: "When I pick you up, we are going to go home and do some crafts together."

When a parent has to be away from a child because of travel, work, or divorce, there are a number of ways to help them hold on when apart. One mother said, "Whenever my kids used to go to their dad's house or away on trips, I would write them notes in envelopes, seal them, and date them. There would be a note for every day." Another mother said that on tough days when the kids really missed their father, who was at work, "we made him a menu on the computer, and then we shopped and bought all the food. Then when he came home for dinner we had everyone take a menu and line up outside the door to enter the 'restaurant.'" Another parent said that when his wife works 12-hour shifts, his three-year-old misses her a lot, so "we make 'Mommy mail' and then leave it in the mailbox. We then text her and tell her to get it when she comes home." When adults help children hang on to the people they love through bridging, it also instills confidence in the caretaker who is available.

BRIDGING THE NIGHTTIME

One of the challenges with the nighttime separation is that there is no caretaker to hand the child off to. Sleep and unconsciousness represent the biggest separation of a child's day, with no one directly caring for them. It is also a time when separation alarm accumulated throughout their day can appear. If a child is facing chronic levels of separation, they may be more stirred up at bedtime.

When Emily and Dan consulted me about Sadie, it was clear she was missing her mother because of her work schedule at night. Fortunately, her mother was able to move around some of her projects and make herself more available at bedtime. This helped decrease Sadie's pursuit of her, fostered a deeper attachment, and reduced some of her separation alarm.

Emily and Dan also worked hard at helping Sadie feel they were connected throughout the night and they were holding on to her. They took the lead in helping her rest, and when Sadie said, "I can't sleep. I'm not tired," they replied with, "Your sleep is not your problem. That's what moms and dads are for." They shifted their posture, and instead of feeling they were being held hostage at night, they started being more generous in their approach. Instead of hurrying and pressuring her to get ready for bed, they went through their bedtime routine trying to convey delight, enjoyment, and warmth. They took the lead in helping her settle, such as turning on the night light before she asked and talking about the plan for the following day as they gave her extra cuddles, kisses, and back rubs. When they left her room, it was for only 5 minutes at a time, and they would return with a paper heart for her to hold on to. Sadie loved the hearts and looked forward to getting one every 5 minutes, 10 minutes, and so on. When Sadie woke up in the morning, she saw a stack of hearts on her bedside table twice as big as before she had gone to sleep. Her parents told her they checked on her throughout the night, and being a preschooler, Sadie believed them!

There are many ways to bridge the night, including tying invisible strings around your beds or between your hearts. You can place pictures of family members in a child's room or place a picture book under their pillow to read in the morning. You can tell them you will meet them in their dreams. For a younger child, it could be helpful for them to sleep with a shirt that smells like Mommy or Daddy to keep them close through the senses. The goal is to take the lead in the attachment dance and point their face into the ways you are holding on to them throughout the night.

Perhaps instead of feeling frustrated as our young children protest going to bed each night, we could fast forward to a time when they won't need us to tuck them in and rub their back, when we won't hear their footsteps running down the hall and their voice telling us they're afraid of monsters. Perhaps we could think about how they will eventually be separated from us as they evolve as independent persons. It would remind our hearts of how hard it is to be apart from someone we love so much. Maybe we could tap into our sadness in seeing them grow up too fast to help us find the generosity they need when they face being alone at night.

3. Matchmaking

Matchmaking is an attachment ritual that cultivates relationships between young children and people in their life. From siblings and grandparents to child care workers, doctors, police officers, and teachers—we need to take the lead in fostering relationships between our children and the people in their attachment village. What young children need most of all is to feel there is an invisible matrix of adults surrounding them for the purpose of caretaking.

Children are creatures of attachment, and their shyness instincts ought to be activated when they are placed in contact with people they do not know—even when they are related to them. A child can be gregarious and talkative at home but retreat and become withdrawn, staying close to their parents, when among strangers. Shyness is not a problem, though it is often perceived as one in contexts where extroverted styles of relating are valued. The shyness instinct is meant to keep children close to their caretakers and prevent others from being able to lead them. It should not feel comfortable for a child to talk to people they don't know and who are not sanctioned by their adults. For example, one father said,

> My three-and-a-half-year-old loves to dance at home and in her class. There was a dance recital at the end of the year where all the parents were invited to watch the kids perform. She refused to dance in front of everyone and just sat on my lap to watch her classmates. I kept telling her to go and dance, but she refused. I didn't want to push her—she is quite sensitive—but I really don't understand why she wouldn't dance when she loves it so much.

The vulnerability of performing in front of strangers was too much for this sensitive child, and the father's response was a generous one.

Gradual entry into daycare and preschool environments is a useful way to introduce someone new to a child. For a child to form a good relationship with their teacher or care provider, making introductions should point out similarities and help them spend time together through an orientation. Matchmaking should point a child's face into an adult attachment as the answer to their separation alarm. Parents can support new relationships by talking kindly about the teacher or caregiver and conveying they sanction the attachment. For example, a mother of a four-year-old entering preschool said,

> My son was anxious about going to preschool, so I jumped at the chance for him to meet the teacher ahead of time and to get to know her better. He brought his favourite books with him, and after I introduced them, I encouraged them to read together. The teacher was great. She told him it was one of her favourite stories too. He also showed her what was in his backpack, and she was interested in anything he had to tell her. It was wonderful to watch them connect.

THREE STEPS TO MATCHMAKING

- **STEP ONE:** Introduce the two parties to each other and set the stage for them to smile and convey a desire to be in each other's presence.

- **STEP TWO:** Prime a connection through drawing attention to something they share in common such as similar likes or preferences.

- **STEP THREE:** Create regular situations, structures, rituals, and traditions where you can bring them together such as holidays, celebrations, meals, gatherings, walks, outings, games, and interactions.

Figure 8.2 Taken from *Neufeld Intensive I: Making Sense of Kids* course

As a child attaches to adults who will care for them, such as grandparents or teachers, their separation alarm should be reduced.

The father of five-year-old Austin used to make a special effort to introduce and matchmake his son to his daycare worker every morning. He would start by telling her he was a king and then say, "I bequeath to you for the day my most prized possession, my first-born heir." He then placed Austin's hand in hers and said to him, "I will pick thee up later and stead thee home to thy castle for nourishment with thy mother. Good day, my son." Austin loved the playful way his father introduced him to his care provider each morning, and it made the separation less alarming.

4. Drawing Out Tears and Cultivating Resilience

When young children are up against an alarming experience they cannot change, the best way forward is to help them find their tears about it. When they are missing their parent at daycare, it is their tears with a caretaker that can help them settle into their home away from home. We don't need to talk children out of their fears, but to help them find ways to express what doesn't work and move to sadness or disappointment.

For a child to find their tears about the separations in their life, they will need the help of an adult who can hold them in the experience of missing until their sadness appears. This will require a trusting relationship with an adult as well as the time and patience to get there. When I witnessed how my children's child care provider was able to comfort other children who missed their parents, I was moved by her compassion. After seeing how gentle and warm she was, I was more comfortable leaving my child in her care. Sadly, another child care provider told me,

> I know young kids need to cry, but it is hard because I worry the parents will judge me and think I am not doing a good job taking care of their child if they are unhappy. I know they miss their

parents, but sometimes I worry if I let them cry, this is all they will do all day. I also know that if I don't let them cry, they are more frustrated and aggressive with each other.

When we have to say goodbye to a young child, it is best to think of it as a one-, two-, three-step dance. It is about giving the child a bridging item to hang onto, greeting the caregiver and ensuring that they can collect the child, and then reminding the child as you leave when you will see them next. The goal is not to torment a child by holding them in a place of separation limbo and drawing out the goodbye. At the same time, it is critical that the child be attached to the adult they are being left with. It takes time to cultivate substitute caretaking relationships, and it is crucial that the adult be able to collect the child and comfort them. The three steps to saying goodbye are guiding principles and not instructions. They are meant to provide an idea as to how to create a predictable structure and routine that can help a young child face connection while separating from a parent.

Adults can reduce the alarm a child experiences at goodbyes by conveying confidence in them that they can handle it. It can be

THREE STEPS TO GOODBYE

- **STEP ONE:** Parent collects the child and gives a bridging object(s) to hang on to such as a picture, note, keychain, necklace.

- **STEP TWO:** Parent greets the caregiver, acts friendly so the child can see a relationship exists between them, and ensures the child is collected by the caregiver.

- **STEP THREE:** Parent tells the child when they will see them next and leaves with a kiss or hug as appropriate.

Figure 8.3 Adapted from *Neufeld Intensive I: Making Sense of Kids* course

helpful to prime them ahead of time and let them know they may feel sad about the separation but they can manage it. For example, many parents are anxious when kindergarten starts but can tell their child, "You might miss me today at school. I will be thinking of you too. I know you will get through this and I will look forward to seeing you later and hearing about your adventures." When picking up a child from school, a parent can invite any sadness in the child by saying, "Did you have any missing in you when you were at school today?" As a child faces separation and is able to shed their sad tears about missing their loved ones, resilience forms as they know they can handle the separation and survive. Young children have a hard time with separation and we shouldn't hold it against them. We need to take the lead in pointing their face into connection every chance we get and to help them find their tears when they are full of missing.

"You're Not the Boss of Me"
Understanding Resistance and Opposition

Whenever you see a board up with "Trespassers
will be prosecuted," trespass at once.
LESLIE STEPHEN,
quoted by his daughter, Virginia Woolf[1]

SUSAN AND CHARLIE were agitated as they spoke to me after a parenting class one evening. Susan said, "We are having a lot of problems toilet training our three-and-a-half-year-old. We started out great, but things have fallen apart. Blake was using the bathroom, but now he refuses. He only wants to wear his diapers." I asked them to tell me more about Blake's resistance. Charlie replied, "We told him he is a big boy now and took away his diapers, but he just goes pee in his underwear." In a panicky voice Susan said, "We need him toilet trained for preschool—they won't take him if he isn't."

I asked them to tell me how things had unfolded, and Susan said, "Whenever he went to the bathroom we praised him and told him he had done a great job. I don't know what happened. Blake just stopped being interested, so we started giving him small rewards." Charlie jumped in: "Now when we tell him to go to the bathroom he pretends he doesn't hear us. We also tried to bribe him. We said we would buy him a bike if he just sat on the toilet, but he refuses."

I asked them a number of questions to determine the root of Blake's resistance, and then replied, "The challenge is Blake is listening to you, but he just isn't obeying. Young children are allergic to coercion, and your desire for toilet training is greater than his. You need to reduce your coercion and create some space for his desire to come back." Susan asked, "How do we do this?" I replied, "I think you need to go back to diapers temporarily. Don't make a big deal of it. Just do it and stop all rewards, praise, punishment, and signs of frustration. When you change his diaper, make it a time of connection where he sees delight, enjoyment, and warmth from you." Both Susan and Charlie looked stunned. Susan said, "Seriously? We need to go backwards?" Charlie replied, "Have you ever changed the diaper of a three-and-a-half-year-old? It's disgusting." I acknowledged that what I was asking seemed counterintuitive but asked if they might give my plan some room and time. Susan said, "I think we have to. We have nothing else left to do—he won't even do this for a bike." She turned to Charlie and said, "You're just going to have to pretend the diapers are full of chocolate pudding." Charlie was clearly not amused.

Susan and Charlie continued to attend the weekly parenting class. I asked them each week how things were going and Charlie shrugged and said, "It's chocolate pudding, Deborah, lots of it." Susan said, "There are no signs of change, but Blake is happy to have his diapers back. I'm trying to collect him and sing to him whenever I change him, kind of like when he was younger." I reaffirmed that they should hold their course and give it time. Three weeks later Susan reported, "I think something is working. He came running into our bedroom at six a.m. yesterday and yelled, 'I have to go poo.' I got the stuff ready to change him, but he looked at me defiantly and said, 'No, I go poo in potty—I do it myself!' and ran to the toilet!" I replied, "His me-do's are coming back—you're on your way now."

Young Children Are Allergic to Coercion

....

WHEN YOU TELL a young child to hurry up, their feet may start to shuffle or stop altogether. You may give them explicit instructions only to find they do the opposite. A mother of a three-year-old said, "Kiefer undid a screw from the bathroom window and I panicked and told him not to lose it. He looked straight at me and threw it outside!" Young children can easily become preoccupied with taboos, so when you tell them not to use "potty" words, they are inclined to keep repeating them. Without any warning they can become disobedient, obstinate, stubborn, resistant, quarrelsome, argumentative, belligerent, incorrigible, noncompliant, and defiant. A mother of a three-year-old said to her daughter, "If you were a dinosaur, you would be the obstreperous kind." True to form, her daughter answered, "No, I wouldn't."

Young children possess an instinct called *counterwill* that can be triggered whenever they feel controlled or coerced by others.[2] By two years of age, they can become sensitive to the wants and wishes of those around them and can respond with resistance. Parents sometimes wonder what happened to their agreeable, complacent, and easygoing child as they begin to erupt in defiance and opposition. A parent of a two-year-old said, "His first response to everything is NO. Even if I ask him if he wants a drink, a cookie, his first response is always NO! He might then immediately change to yes, but no comes first. If he needs to be in his car seat, he will say no then scream NO! He will still scream, even if cajoled, persuaded, or offered a treat." A child's resistance can be interpreted as being on purpose or manipulative, or as intentionally trying to push a parent's buttons when they are only being true to their counterwill instinct. The ability to say "no" may be problematic for adults, but it is a developmental achievement that ought to be celebrated too.

The instinct to resist and oppose is one of the most misunderstood dynamics in adult–child relationships. Counterwill is not a learned response but an emotional reaction that plays a critical role in preserving the self and becoming a separate person. Young children are allergic to other people's agendas because they are still trying to figure out their own, hence their favourite line—"I do it myself." The more a child develops their own will, the less they will feel compelled to resist and counter the will of others. Counterwill in young children stems from their undeveloped will that is still maturing. It takes a lifetime to understand one's own values, goals, and motives. For a young child, making sense of their own preferences, wants, wishes, priorities, and decisions is what happens when they are at rest and playing. Young children won't outgrow these instincts when they have a more coherent self, just outgrow the need to operate out of them.

The challenge is, nothing pushes an adult's buttons like a resistant child, especially if the parent has a strong agenda or will of their own. Everyday agendas can become trigger points for counterwill reactions from a young child: getting dressed, going to sleep, using the toilet, brushing their teeth or hair, and eating healthy. A grandparent eager for her four-year-old grandson to try her homemade pumpkin pie was told, "No, sorry, I don't eat pumpkin pie, Oma. I'm a vegetarian." When young children defy adult wishes, it can lead to a battle of wills with ferocious power struggles ensuing. One father said, "I heard my wife arguing with my three-year-old in the bathroom. She wanted her to get out of the bath, but Lauren didn't want to. They went around in circles with each one digging in until I finally broke it up." Engaging in counterwill battles with a young child can leave a parent filled with regret, as this parent discovered:

> When my daughter was about 5, we were going out to a very fancy
> restaurant with our extended family for a special celebration. I told
> her that she had to dress up. At this age, she loved nothing better
> than to dress up, so I thought she would relish the opportunity. No!
> I did not know about counterwill then. She was indignant that she

"had" to dress up and that a restaurant could dictate what people wear and that she didn't have any say in the matter. I thought she was simply being belligerent, and all of a sudden I was questioning everything about my parenting, worrying that I had been way too lax with her, that she wouldn't follow such a simple direction. And I was frustrated! I thought I must need to be firmer—much firmer. Well, you can imagine the battle of counterwills that ensued as I insisted even more firmly that she had to do as I asked. I would have saved us both lots of angst and grief that night had I only known about counterwill.

Some parents react strongly to a child's defiance, believing that if they don't it will only lead to further disobedience. When adults push for compliance at all costs or try to extinguish resistant behaviour, the instinctive and emotional reasons for a child's opposition are missed, shamed, or thwarted. The belief that resistance and opposition must be unlearned (a) doesn't recognize or value the developmental benefits of having one's own mind and (b) fails to appreciate that we need to grow a child out of resistance, not punish or teach a child to behave otherwise. An adult can make a child capitulate to their demands with enough force, but this often leads to resentment and confusion, and erodes attachment. Psychoanalyst Otto Rank, who wrote extensively about counterwill, said that parental overreactions to it were one of the biggest causes of insecurity in a child.[3] To preserve a relationship with a young child, we need to understand how counterwill serves development, how to avoid provoking it, and how to deal with it when we do.

Forms of Coercion and Control

THE BELIEF THAT young children won't do anything unless they are coerced conveys little faith in a child's inherent desire to be good for their adults. It doesn't take into account the power of attachment and how young children will naturally follow the people they are connected to. As a result, adults mistakenly use physical, behavioural, emotional, and cognitive forms of control and coercion to push for compliance rather than leaning on attachment strategies.

Adults may *physically* move a child by picking them up or pushing them along. This is easier to do when a child is small but more difficult as they get bigger. A child can meet physical coercion with thrashing, screaming, or going limp. When one father grabbed his five-year-old son in a football hold and ran out of a restaurant, the child started screaming, "Help! Help! Someone help me. I'm being abducted!" When children are forced in one direction, you can predict a counterforce in the opposite.

Negative reinforcement is a form of *behavioural* coercion aimed at reducing the likelihood that certain actions will be repeated. However, when a young child is told that they will be in trouble or that certain behaviours are off limits, it can actually increase the likelihood that they will behave that way. For example, in the classic forbidden-toy study, researchers gave children either a severe or mild threat against playing with a toy.[4] The more severe the threat, the more a child desired to play with it, despite warnings. The child remains unaware of this instinct and simply acts without understanding when told *not* to do something. A parent told me, "When I was in kindergarten, my mother told me not to show people my underwear before I went onstage for my Christmas concert. Before I knew it, I was standing there with my skirt pulled over my head, showing the audience my underwear."

Behavioural forms of coercion also include positive reinforcement, by which a child is rewarded or praised so as to encourage similar behaviours. Many people miss how controlling a reward can feel to a young child, probably because rewards are seen as being positive. Rewards, however, reveal the desires of others, which can trump and diminish a child's own intentions. A classic study on motivation in young children found that those who were praised for using magic markers were less interested in playing with them than were those who were not rewarded.[5] Alfie Kohn, the author of *Punished by Rewards*, states that extrinsic rewards are short-lived and diminish a child's internal motivation.[6] Rewards given to achieve compliance can interfere with a child's natural desire to learn or genuinely care about others.

Emotional forms of coercion include shaming a child or trying to make them feel guilty for their impulses and immature actions. Adults use a child's emotions to control their behaviour with statements such as "If you were a good brother, you would stop hitting your sister," "If you loved your mom, you would help her pick up the toys," and "See what Eva did? Isn't she a good friend for helping out?" Emotionally coercive statements imply that there is something fundamentally wrong with the child. Emotional coercion not only wounds a child's relationship with an adult but creates a shaming environment.

Cognitive forms of coercion include telling a child what to think and believe; agreement with an adult becomes a form of obedience. Young children should naturally be driven to make sense of their world and form their own meanings about it. For example, a four-year-old girl told her brother, "Did you know you have taste bugs on your tongue?" She also told him, "There are cutlery worms in the garden and they eat all the vegetables. That's why there are holes in them." Another four-year-old told his father, "I have goosebumps on my forehead." When his father discounted his experience by correcting the fact with "You only get those on your arms and legs when you are excited or scared," the little boy said, "Fine, they're chickenpox, then."

The Two Faces of Counterwill

THE COUNTERWILL INSTINCT is critical in the development of a child in two ways: (1) it protects attachment by resisting outside influence and direction and (2) it prepares the way for separate functioning and independence. It is important to note that there are other reasons why a young child may be resistant, such as fear, anxiety, anger, frustration, hostility, and mistrust. Noncompliance can also result from dysfunction, curiosity, forgetfulness, or lack of understanding, rather than from the counterwill instinct. Before dealing with a child's resistance and opposition, it is helpful to consider how it has been provoked.

1. **Counterwill Protects Attachment**
   The counterwill instinct preserves a parent's rightful place in a child's life as being the one to lead and take care of them. Young children should not be amenable to being bossed around by just anyone; this is why they are resistant to strangers. A mother of two young children asked me about an incident:

   > When I was in a store shopping, this grandmother came over and tried to talk to my kids in a friendly way. She was telling them how cute they were and asking their names and how old they were. She didn't mean any harm, but my eldest, age 4, stuck out his tongue and gave her a nasty face. He then went and hid behind my legs and wouldn't look at her anymore. I was so embarrassed. I just told the grandma he was shy, but I am wondering why he acted this way.

THE COUNTERWILL INSTINCT

1) is a defensive reaction to perceived control and coercion
2) serves attachment by protecting against outside influence and direction
3) serves development by preparing the way for separate functioning

The first step in finding one's own WILL is to resist and counter the WILL of others.

Figure 9.1 Taken from Neufeld *Making Sense of Counterwill* course

Counterwill is a natural attachment instinct that prevents a child from being influenced and directed by people their parents have not sanctioned as part of their attachment village.

This raises the question of why children are resistant to a parent's direction when there is an existing relationship between them. Resistance to a parent stems from a lack of brain integration in young children—they can attach to only one person or thing at a time. If a parent gives them a direction or command without engaging their attachment instincts, the child can feel coerced and controlled, thereby eliciting a counterwill response. For example, if a young child is engaged in play alone or with a peer or sibling, their attachment instincts are not focused on their parent. A father of a two-and-a-half- and a four-year-old relayed the following story:

> My wife told me to get the kids, who were watching TV, to come for dinner. They didn't even look at me or acknowledge I was there, so I just turned the TV off. Well, that got their attention. They started screaming, "No! Don't turn it off," and "Turn it on!" I told them it was time for dinner and they yelled, "No! We don't want dinner." My wife then yelled at me, "Did you collect them before you directed them? You need to collect them before you tell them what to do!" At this point, I had three people yelling at me. It was brutal. I told my wife later she hadn't collected me before she started telling me what to do either.

Collecting a child is one of the best ways to engage their attachment instincts and involves getting in their face in a friendly way and getting their eyes or perhaps a smile (as discussed in chapter 4). It is important to collect young children before giving them commands, obligations, expectations, or demands or pressuring them to do something, as their default mode is one of resistance. Attachment is what renders a young child amenable to our caretaking and makes them more agreeable to complying with our wishes, wanting to please us, deferring, measuring up, and being good for us. In short, counterwill and attachment have a teeter-totter relationship. When attachment is strong, counterwill is weak or nonexistent. When attachment is weak, counterwill reactions will be strong.

What could this father have done to collect his kids? First, a screen is a formidable distraction given it can hold a child's attention and stimulate them. To collect their attention, the father would need a prior working relationship with the kids. He would need to come alongside them, perhaps ask them what they were watching, try to get their eyes, or engage them in some way by sharing an interest in the show for a couple of minutes. If he was able to get their attention and they protested coming for dinner, he would probably have to make some room for tears around their disappointment. If the father repeatedly found he couldn't collect their attention and engage their attachment instincts, it would be important to consider if there was a relational problem between him and the children.

COUNTERWILL PROBLEMS EXIST WHEN THERE ARE ATTACHMENT PROBLEMS

When a young child's counterwill seems to be more chronic and enduring than fluid, it may be indicative of a relational problem. There are a number of attachment problems that render a child resistant to taking directions from their adults, including peer orientation and alpha issues (see chapters 4 and 5).

Further attachment issues that foster counterwill problems in young children include not having a relationship with the adults who are in charge of them. If children are not attached to their daycare, preschool, or kindergarten teachers, their default mode of relating will be counterwill. The adult's title or "role" in the child's life has no influence on whether the child is actually attached to that adult. An aunt taking care of her five-year-old niece said, "I asked her to help me put away the toys and she said no and told me I wasn't the boss of her. I told her she needed to come and eat and she refused again. I reminded her that I was her aunt, but it made little difference to her." Counterwill problems will exist wherever there are attachment issues.

Another attachment problem is not having a deep enough relationship with an adult to weaken the counterwill instinct. Sometimes children are attached too superficially, through senses, sameness, or belonging, which doesn't give their caretakers strong enough influence over a child. Furthermore, if a child's emotions have become stuck and there are few signs of vulnerable feelings, their development can be delayed, making them more prone to counterwill responses because of immaturity.

When a child gets stuck in counterwill reactions, they are more likely to face increasing coercion and control by adults in their life. In turn, they will feel increasingly pushed and therefore will be more resistant. When a child gets locked into resisting, adults can get stuck in pushing, which further erodes the relationship. The child is usually seen as being the one with the resistance problem and may be labelled oppositional, noncompliant, or defiant. What gets missed is *why* a young child is not attached to the adults in their life.

When attachment problems have rendered a child stuck in their counterwill responses, that child is no longer motivated to be loyal to, measure up for, attend and listen to, look up to, or make things work for their adult. They will orient negatively to the parent and will work to rule, defy, counter, annoy, or irritate. The only way to

THE CYCLE OF STUCK COUNTERWILL

A tragedy in three acts

- **ACT I:** When kids get stuck, adults start pushing.
- **ACT II:** When kids feel pushed, they put on the brakes.
- **ACT III:** When kids get stuck in their resistance, adults tend to get stuck in their persistence.

Figure 9.2 Adapted from Neufeld *Making Sense of Counterwill* course

change these responses is for the adult to lead by cultivating a stronger relationship and not let themselves be alienated. Bridging the problematic behaviour and retreating from dealing with incidents are two strategies that can help prevent further wounding to their relationship as well. (See chapter 10.)

2. Counterwill Prepares the Way for Separate Functioning and Independence

Counterwill is a natural defence against the will of others to make way for the child to discover their own preferences, wants, wishes, goals, and aspirations. Children need an invitation for attachment, and they also need an invitation to become their own person. A parent told me, "My mother and I had a great relationship until I turned three and got my own mind. She couldn't handle me having an agenda that differed from hers, so we just struggled from that day onward."

The characteristics a young child exhibits that make them difficult to care for are the same ones we will long for as they become adults—saying no, disagreeing, and having their own ideas, plans, and purpose. It doesn't work to encourage our children to have their own mind only when it doesn't contradict ours. At the same time, adults need to lead and be responsible for taking care of children.

Children need to be born psychologically, and counterwill creates a womb where a self can grow and boundaries can form. Selfhood is a process of increasing integration, of merging thoughts and feelings together to form a "ME." Although growth into selfhood is critical to development, it is not inevitable and occurs spontaneously after approximately three years of fulfilling attachment. This growth is evident when we start to hear a child say, "me-do" or "I do it myself." Pediatrician Donald Winnicott wrote that when a child is able to identify themselves in terms of "I AM" language, a critical phase in human development has unfolded.[7] Counterwill is meant to protect a child's emerging self against other people's ideas, agendas, intentions, judgements, expectations, demands, values, and desires. Strong counterwill responses are designed to be transitional as the emergent self grows. Starting at the age of 2, a young child's counterwill responses can be brazen and untempered, but as a child gets older and starts to develop mixed feelings, they will have more self-control over their responses.

While I was at the park with my kids one day, my friend asked me to watch her three-year-old while she attended to another child. Simon was trying desperately to climb onto a duck that rocked back and forth on a big metal spring. As he struggled, I moved in to help him, but he looked at me sternly and said, "No, I do!" I backed away and gave Simon more space to struggle, but I was still able to reach him if he needed me. He struggled some more but looked at me again and saw I hadn't moved enough for his liking. He charged at me with his fists and pushed me away from his duck. His mother saw him and told him to stop pushing me. I jumped in and told her Simon had just wanted to get on the duck all by himself and I had merely been in his way. What Simon couldn't say was, "I am in the midst of my individuation and differentiation as a separate being and your will is impeding mine from developing further." Without language and insight, three-year-olds will use whatever means they have to get their instinctive counterwill messages across.

In reflecting on Susan and Charlie's toilet-training troubles, it is clear that their agenda had become bigger than Blake's when it came to being diaper free. They had praised and rewarded him when he acted in accordance with their plans, but this left little room for Blake's desires or interests to lead the way. His "want-to's" became his "have-to's," and instead of using his initiative to try something new, he felt the weight of his parents' expectations. Where he could have been helped to find his own purpose and meanings in leaving his diapers behind, he felt pressure and directives. His interest in using the toilet was trumped by incentives, diminishing his desire to "do it myself." The more resistance Blake put up, the more persistent his parents became, escalating counterwill reactions on both sides. When Susan and Charlie took a tactical retreat into attaching with him and stopped all pressure, Blake's emergent self led the way and he began using the toilet again. The strategy with young children is to avoid letting them see or feel when our agendas are bigger than theirs, especially when we need their cooperation—like in sleeping, eating, dressing, toilet training, and daily hygiene tasks.

When a child is emerging as a separate being, they will be curious, want to try new things, think for themselves, see options and choices in life, want to be different, and seek independence. We need not to push or thrust a child towards autonomy but to allow natural counterwill instincts to prepare the way. When a child sees they have options and can make choices, they should naturally start to feel responsible for these, along with feeling guilt about how their actions affect others. We don't need to force these lessons on our children; healthy growth and development will pave the way for responsible functioning to unfold. As a child's will develops and fortifies in the adolescent years, they should feel both the freedom and the autonomy this brings as well as the moral responsibility and guilt inherent in being a separate person.

Distinguishing between the Two Faces of Counterwill

PARENTS OFTEN WONDER how to distinguish between the two forms of counterwill. The key issue to consider is *what came before* the counterwill response. If a child's attachment instincts were not actively engaged before a parent tried to direct them, then counterwill is resulting from the parent not having enough relational influence. For example, one parent ran into trouble because she hadn't collected her son before trying to get him to join her in leaving the house:

My son was playing with his planes when I told him we needed to put away his toys so we could leave to pick up his sister from kindergarten. He ignored me until I raised my voice and told him to get his shoes on because we had to leave. He yelled, "No!" so I moved closer and he started saying "No no no no no" and pushed me away. So I got his shoes and tried to put them on, but he kept kicking his legs, making it impossible. I finally decided to take him out in the stroller without his shoes because he was just too difficult.

If the parent had seen her son's reaction as counterwill, she might have been able to take a tactical retreat instead of battling him. She could have moved to collect him before proceeding to get his shoes on.

If a counterwill response came *after* a time of fulfilling attachment with a child, then it is probably in the service of helping them becoming their own person. For example, a mother of a three-and-a-half-year-old was surprised by her daughter's resistance one morning:

I had collected Jessica, read her books, and talked about our day. When I went to get her dressed, she became really resistant. Instead of being agreeable like she had been, Jessica looked at me and started saying, "No, I don't like that shirt." She went through all of the shirts in her drawer, choosing one and then changing her mind, back and forth. It was terrible. When I said to her, "Come on, let me help you get dressed," she turned to me and said, "No, lady, I do it all by myself!" Sometimes her Jekyll-and-Hyde nature baffles me.

In this case, Jessica was fulfilled, and her emergent, albeit immature, self began to come forth. What is true in both examples of counterwill is that there is nothing like a young child's resistance to baffle, confuse, and defy all adult logic.

Strategies for Dealing with Counterwill
Resistance and Opposition

. . . .

THE SECRET TO handling counterwill is to not take it personally—a seemingly impossibly tall order when a parent's own counterwill has been activated. Young children routinely come to a standstill as part of daily life. The key is for adults to lead through the impasses without disrupting the connection. The challenge lies in not reacting by using more force and leverage to control a child; this will only exacerbate their resistance and/or harm the relationship.

Depending on what has provoked the counterwill response, there are three strategies that can be used to diffuse and manage resistance and opposition in young children: (1) bridging counterwill and increasing attachment, (2) reducing coercion and control, and (3) making room for the child's will.

1. Bridging Counterwill and Increasing Attachment

One of the most critical things to convey in the midst of counterwill reactions is that the relationship is still intact despite the resistance. Adults need to find a way to maintain an alpha position when they are faced with a child's resistance, without forcing their will on a child. A number of strategies are helpful in bridging the problematic behaviour and holding on to the relationship:

- *Don't use separation as a consequence.* Attachment is a child's greatest need, so using time-outs or taking away possessions or privileges is bound to be provocative. These actions will probably increase a child's resistance and add frustration as well as alarm to the mix.

- *Anticipate and expect counterwill.* Given that young children are immature and lack a fully formed self, counterwill reactions should be anticipated and expected when dealing with them. The goal is to interpret their actions not as personal, intentional, or manipulative but as instinctive and emotionally driven. Although we may not understand what underlies their resistance, if we expect it, we may be less likely to overreact and be alienated by it.

- *Don't make behaviour the bottom line.* When children resist, adults often demand they change their behaviour before anything else is allowed to proceed. This serves to increase a child's resistance and exacerbate their reaction. For example, if a child refuses to get their shoes on and a parent responds with demands that this happens before anything else does, both sides are likely to get stuck in their own counterwill reaction.

- *Reflect the resistance as natural and normal.* When a young child is resistant and oppositional, coming alongside and acknowledging that they feel controlled or coerced can diffuse their reaction. For example, a parent may say, "Yes, I know you don't like it sometimes when I tell you what to do." This doesn't mean the adult has to drop their agenda, only that they acknowledge that the child may have a different one from theirs.

- *Keep reactions to counterwill in check.* The more an adult sees themselves as in charge and responsible for a child, the more provocative a child's counterwill can feel. A father said, "I just feel like I have to squash my children's spirits when they are resistant and defiant so they won't behave like this as an adult." It is frustrating, even infuriating, for a parent to be defied. Counterwill in a child is provocative, and the answer lies in not responding to them from this place. When a parent can hold on to their caring for a child and their concern for the relationship, it should help temper their reaction and lead the way towards patience and tolerance. It is important to find a way to lead through the impasses with everyone's dignity intact.

- *Repair damage done by counterwill overreactions.* When you have over-reacted to a child's counterwill, repairing the relationship is the first order of business. This may involve taking the lead in apologizing and assuming responsibility for your actions. If a child is still feeling hurt after an apology, then letting them know you are okay with them being upset is important too. Emotional overreactions by parents, such as crying or pleading for forgiveness, will court alpha problems in a child as they assume responsibility for an adult's feelings. The goal is to touch the relationship bruise, take responsibility for it, and move on with the business of taking care of them. Parenting isn't about being perfect but about taking responsibility for our imperfections and proceeding from there.

Bridging counterwill reactions in young children requires patience, faith, and a belief that the more a child grows as a separate self, the less they will need to operate out of their counterwill instinct. In the meantime, our best measure is to maintain an alpha presence and not allow their behaviour to break our connection.

When it comes to counterwill responses in young children, adults need to see themselves as the ones responsible for leading children out of the impasse. Changing the subject or postponing the discussion can achieve this, as can giving the reaction some time and space until it dissipates. It is important not to identify the child with their resistant reactions, with statements such as "Why are you so stubborn?" or "No one wants to be with you if you act like this." Coming alongside their feelings of being controlled or coerced will avoid shaming them for something that comes naturally. There are also times when a parent must use their alpha stance to hold a child in some upset to help them realize that resistance is sometimes futile.

If a child's resistance stems from a weak relationship with an adult, then cultivating a stronger attachment will be the first task. Before taking care of a child, an adult should ensure they can collect them, indicating they have enough attachment power to do their job. Strengthening the relationship can be achieved through the expression of delight, enjoyment, and warmth as well as through connecting through sameness, belonging and loyalty, significance, or whatever other means they are attaching.

2. Reducing Coercion and Control

Reducing the amount of control and coercion a child experiences in the following ways can help prevent counterwill reactions as well as deal with them when they arise:

- *Refrain from using a commanding or prescriptive manner.* When adults give directions to young children, they often change their tone in anticipation of being resisted. Directions tend to come across as more forceful or commanding, increasing the likelihood of a counterwill response.

- *Make agendas less explicit.* Adults can be very explicit when they give directions to young children. For example, a parent might say, "Get your shoes and coat on. We are leaving for school and I don't want to be late for work." The direct and forceful nature of this request can easily provoke counterwill in a young child, whereas a more implicit approach would be less provocative. For example, instead of telling them to hurry up and get ready, a parent might focus on the plan for the day while they put a child's jacket and shoes on: "Your teacher told me you are going to have a special visitor for show and tell at preschool today. Do you know who it might be?" By making the adult's agenda less obvious, fewer counterwill reactions may occur. And making something playful is a sure way to reduce coercion and make a parent's agenda less explicit.

- *Refrain from focusing on the* SHOULDS, *the* MUSTS, *and the* HAVE-TO's. Some of the most commanding statements a child hears include *should, must,* or *have to.* These phrases bait counterwill responses by suggesting that anything else will not be tolerated. Furthermore, they erode a child's want-to's and intrinsic motivation, crushing their emerging spirits, which are eager to learn and try new things.

- *Use as little force and leverage as possible.* Physical, behavioural, emotional, and cognitive forms of coercion will exacerbate counterwill reactions and create an adversarial relationship. Sometimes adults are loath to give up their negative and positive reinforcement tools, clinging to them in the hope these will render a child more amenable. What is lost is an awareness that attachment is the context in which children are most amenable to following their adults, bending to their will, and sharing their values.

- *Back off until you have a better attachment hold.* One of the most effective strategies when a counterwill reaction has been provoked is to temporarily back off until attachment instincts are activated. When faced with resistance, an adult might say, "I am going to let you think about this and I'll come back in a minute," or "I have changed my mind. I will give you another five minutes to play and then we are leaving." It is important to convey that you are not alienated by their resistance or displaced from your alpha role. For example, one mother said her daughter turned to her on a preschool outing to a farm and asserted, "The more you tell me not to touch the donkey, the more I am going to." Luckily, the group moved on to tour another animal pen, and instead of addressing her behaviour directly, the mother collected her daughter and gave her a snack. After collecting her, the mother solicited good intentions from her (see chapter 10 on discipline) about listening to the directions she was given.

- *Use structures and routines to orchestrate behaviour.* Given that young children are allergic to coercion and control, structure and routine are wonderful ways to bring order to their behaviour without having to "boss them around." I was always amazed at how my children's preschool teacher could employ structure and routine to signal circle time, play, and snack time. She would start to sing a clean-up song that alerted the kids to the transition away from play and into outdoor time—but not before they picked up their toys.

- *Draw attention AWAY from the coercive elements of the situation.* The more coercive a situation is, the more you want to draw attention away from the elements that would provoke counterwill. Seatbelts, strollers, and shopping carts all constrain children and routinely provoke counterwill. Instead of allowing their focus to go to the constraining elements, a parent could talk to the child, sing songs, or feed them. One of the times children can feel coerced is at the dinner table, where they are expected to sit and eat. The more the focus is on eating their food, the more counterwill can be provoked. Making mealtime less coercive and directing their attention to stories, fun, or just engaging with the family around something other than food can draw their eyes away from what is most coercive in this setting. The more you say, "Eat your vegetables," the less they will want to eat them.

3. **Making Room for the Child's Will**
   When a child's counterwill reaction stems from a move towards independent functioning, giving them room to exert their own will is a useful strategy. This can be achieved in a number of ways, but it is important not to put them in charge of any caretaking or decision making regarding their relational needs.

- *Provide some sense of choice.* When a young child is resistant to a parent's agenda, giving them some choice or wiggle room to flex their own mind helps them feel less coerced. For example, when going to bed, they could choose what pyjamas they want to wear, what book they want to read, what toothbrush they want to use, or what song they want you to sing to them.

- *Put the focus on the child's will.* Helping a child discover their own will and placing emphasis on their own desires, goals, reasons, and meanings will help reduce counterwill. For example, a parent might say, "You just want everyone to stop telling you what to do. You want to have your own mind about this." It doesn't mean the child gets their way, but it validates that they have a will of their own. A parent of a four-year-old said he was teaching his daughter how to fold clothes but she resisted his direction and said, "I have my own way of folding my clothes," and her father was happy to indulge her.

- *Make room for the child's initiative and involvement.* To reduce counterwill, invite a child to be involved or take initiative in participating in an activity. For example, one mother was trying to help her three-year-old put animal faces on balloons cut out of construction paper. In her eagerness to help, the mother started telling her daughter where to put the animal body parts and how it should look. Her daughter lost all interest and refused to do the craft. Instead, at playtime a child could choose what they want to do, or at the arts and crafts table they could decide how they want to use the supplies in front of them.

- *Solicit good intentions where possible.* When a child's cooperation is important, soliciting their good intentions ahead of time can be helpful in preventing counterwill. Soliciting good intentions requires engaging a child's attachment instincts and using the relationship to ask them to cooperate with a set of guidelines for behaviour. The child's agreement helps to avoid resistant behaviours in particular situations. For example, a parent had to take her children to their father's workplace in a highly professional environment. Instead of waiting to direct and command appropriate behaviour while at his workplace and thus risk opposition, she solicited the children's good intentions for behaviour ahead of time. She asked them if she could count on them to behave, "and not to run, scream, or act silly at Daddy's work today." She said a number of people commented and were surprised at how well behaved the children were.

· *Place them in charge where appropriate and possible.* Young children need to have areas in which they can be in charge, exercise their own will, and develop their own preferences (with the exception of anything to do with their attachment needs). Parents need to find places, things, or activities children can have control over, such as playtime, learning a new skill, or getting dressed. One parent put her daughter in charge of getting herself dressed, with particular guidelines such as no dress-up clothes outside and no pyjamas in the daytime. Beth started to dress herself, and at the age of 4 she was pretty proud of her efforts. She would parade her outfits for the family to see and asked her uncle one day what he thought about her ensemble. He responded honestly and told her he wasn't sure fuchsia and red went together, to which she replied, "Oh yes they do."

Counterwill protects a young child from following people they are not attached to and paves the way for a separate self to emerge. Sometimes children's resistance stems from adults not activating their attachment instincts before directing them, whereas it could also mean children are just trying to figure things out for themselves. It is important to read a child and consider what came before their resistance and then determine how best to proceed. Although a young child's "me-do's" may seem insignificant, they are the building blocks for growth into personhood. In adolescence, they will use their "me-do's" to cross the bridge from childhood into adulthood. The challenge for adults who raise young children is to make room for their "me-do's" today, for they hold the promises of "ME" tomorrow.

Maturity Is the Answer to Immature Behaviour

ADULTS WANT MATURE, well-behaved children and believe discipline will get them there—but it won't. Discipline is what adults do to impose order on the disorder of immaturity. Discipline is how adults intervene and compensate for the maturity that is missing. Adults need to use discipline to buy a child time to grow up. Adults need to assume responsibility for pointing a child in a civilized direction but give them room to get there. They will need to hold on to their relationship in spite of infractions, use insight to deal with what has stirred a child up, and help children understand their emotional world better. A kindergarten teacher told her student, "Tessa, you need to work on being more mature, such as saying goodbye to your mother without being upset." Her mother replied, "Tessa will be more mature when she matures."

There is a developmental plan that leads to maturity, bringing social and emotional responsibility with it. Advice on "what to do" with immature behaviour has become divorced from a broader developmental agenda that considers what conditions children *need* in order to grow as separate, social, and adaptive beings. The topic of discipline has become a jumble of superficial solutions, isolated directions, and contradictory answers. Discipline advice has morphed into discussions about teachable moments, strategies for achieving compliance, and instructions for how to get young kids to control themselves. Parents are given prescriptions for discipline without understanding how methods work, the limitations to their effectiveness, and potential risks to development. One parent I knew read every discipline book she could find and engaged with her children differently each week. As her discipline techniques changed, her kids were less convinced she knew how to take care of them.

Part of the problem with discipline today is it is largely based on behavioural and learning approaches that aim to extinguish behaviour rather than understand its source. Good behaviour is rewarded or praised, and bad behaviour is punished. Emotional expression is treated as a problem rather than understood as having a job to do in solving a problem for a child. Resistance is seen as something to be suppressed rather than as stemming from the counterwill instinct that preserves selfhood. Tantrums are treated as fires that need to be put out, routinely stoking the frustration that gave rise to them. Attention problems are seen as deficits in the child instead of as characteristics of an immature system that can focus on only one thing at a time. In short, behaviour is treated at face value, with the emotions and instincts underpinning it eclipsed. The focus of discipline has become myopically focused on providing the right consequences to shape behaviour into a mature form. These methods miss the big developmental picture altogether—discipline is what we do while waiting for maturity to unfold.

B.F. Skinner suggested that the secret to having good children was to deprive them of approval and make approval conditional upon compliance. Good behaviour was rewarded with praise or parental closeness, whereas bad behaviour led to punishment and separation. Contemporary discipline takes a similar approach and uses temporary withdrawal of affection through time-outs or separation to achieve good behaviour. Simply put, a parent's love is used as a tool to shape behaviour—a child is invited to be close when they are good and sent away when they are not. A child is made to work for love and approval by meeting parental demands, negating any chance for true rest. These disciplinary practices have become the norm, but they erode relationships and create emotional distress in young children.[2]

A different approach is needed if parents are to offer a child a generous invitation to rest in their care, are to unlock the capacity for play, and are to foster conditions conducive to growth. Discipline strategies need to use the power of attachment to bring a child into orbit around an adult. Adults are the ones who need to provide order, keep young children safe, and give directions when they are impulsive, egocentric, and inconsiderate. As one parent said, "My focus used to be on 'He is so rude,' but now I see 'He is so frustrated right now.' What I focus on informs my next step, and focusing on the emotion seems to point me in the right direction." Attachment-safe and developmentally friendly discipline protects and preserves a child's soft heart as well as their right relationships with adults.

The Six Traits of Well-Behaved Children*

THE SIX TRAITS associated with well-behaved children cannot be taught and must be grown. Well-behaved children (a) want to be good, (b) are easily alarmed, (c) feel futility, (d) are appropriately attached to adults, (e) are well intentioned, and (f) are well tempered. As a child develops these traits, they become easier to care for and more mature in their behaviour and emotional responses. If a child doesn't outgrow the preschooler personality by ages 5 to 7, or 7 to 9 for sensitive kids, and continues to have behaviour problems, attention should go to considering which of these traits are missing and why. When these traits are absent, there is no amount of discipline that will fix the resulting problems or restore healthy development.

Children should *want to be good* for the people they are attached to and resist orders from those they are not. The desire to be good stems from deep fulfilling attachments with adults who collect them regularly and provide a generous invitation for rest, as discussed in chapters 4 and 5. The challenge for young children is that their lack of self-control prevents them from consistently actualizing their desires to be good.

Well-behaved children also have a *healthy alarm system* that moves them to caution when facing danger or when they are told to keep out of harm's way. Good alarm systems make children conscientious and concerned about their actions. For an alarm system to function

---

* Gordon Neufeld, "Theoretical construct on the six traits of well-behaved children," *Making Sense of Discipline*, course, Neufeld Institute, Vancouver, BC (2011).

properly, a child must be able to feel afraid and be free of emotional defences. The alarm system will become crippled when vulnerable feelings are defended against, which is sometimes the case in peer-oriented and alpha children.

Well-behaved children also *feel futility* when they are up against the things they cannot change, as discussed in chapter 7. They can adapt to not getting their way, accept another's decisions, and adjust to the limits and restrictions in their life. A child should become increasingly adaptive from the ages of 2 to 6, as the futilities of life are presented to them and support is given in finding their tears. The adaptive process requires soft hearts and emotions to be felt in a vulnerable way. If a child's tears are stuck and emotional defences are present, the child's adaptive capacity will be diminished or missing altogether.

Well-behaved children are *appropriately attached* to the people who are responsible for them. These adults serve as role models and represent the values that will help them fit into society in a productive way. Parents need to assume responsibility for matchmaking a child to people in their attachment village, as discussed in chapter 8. These adults should share similar values so as to prevent pulling the child out of their orbit around a parent. If a child is peer oriented, there

---

SIX TRAITS OF WELL-BEHAVED CHILDREN

1) They **WANT TO BE GOOD** for those responsible for them.
2) They can see trouble coming and are appropriately moved to caution **(EASILY ALARMED)**.
3) They can **FEEL FUTILITY** when it is encountered.
4) Their socializing attachments are appropriate **(APPROPRIATELY ATTACHED)**.
5) They have their own goals and agendas **(WELL-INTENTIONED)**.
6) They are able to think twice when experiencing troublesome impulses **(WELL-TEMPERED)**.

Figure 10.1 Taken from Neufeld *Discipline That Doesn't Divide* course

will be little desire to be good or follow the adults responsible for them. They will aim to please friends instead, often at the expense of adult rules and guidelines. A parent will need to restore their relationship with their child in order to influence their behaviour.

Children who are well behaved are able to form their own goals and agendas through *good intentions*. Counterwill, discussed in chapter 9, and play, from chapter 3, are important instincts that pave the way for this growth. When a sense of self has developed, a child should move to independent functioning, assuming responsibility for their own actions. The development of personal intentions rests on having fulfilling attachments, which bring release from relational hunger. Parents can use a child's own intentions to point them in the direction of civilized behaviour.

Children who are well behaved are also *tempered* and have self-control as a result of prefrontal brain integration, as discussed in chapter 2. At this time, a child will be able to consider the needs of others before responding, think twice before acting on their emotions, and mix feelings and thoughts. The capacity for patience, forgiveness, and perseverance will be unlocked along with a coherent sense of self. The impulsive, egocentric, and inconsiderate ways of the young child should become tempered, helping them actualize their desires for good behaviour.

The answer to why children are well behaved is that the natural developmental plan has unfolded as it should. There is a plan for good behaviour, and we need to put our trust in this. As one parent wrote,

This is such a complete shift from a focus on behaviour and working on the behaviour directly. I so appreciate the fact that nature has a vital role and that as a parent, I am not responsible to grow the child up. As a young parent, I did not know this. I truly thought it was up to me to "nip it in the bud," to "be on top of every little problem." I was so uptight as a parent because I really was invested in good behaviour. I didn't understand the spontaneous nature of growing up.

Critique of Current Discipline Practices

THREE OF THE most popular approaches to discipline use attachment alarm to get a child to change their behaviour. Although they may seem successful in getting a child to stop acting a certain way, they often do so by trading on a child's most important need. As a result, alarm-, separation-, and consequence-based forms of discipline can create emotional and relational distress in young children. There are alternative ways to deal with incidents with young children, but these have become lost in the pressure for compliance and mature behaviour. As one child care provider said,

> I think this "consequence" thinking is so incongruent with parents' intuition that they have to go blind to be able to follow through. They believe they are doing the right thing, they are driven from a place of love and care for their children, yet this is not loving behaviour. The real difficulties start when these methods don't work anymore, but the parents don't know what to do and feel desperate.

1. **Alarm-Based Methods**

   A child's alarm system is designed to move them to caution when facing threat or danger. Discipline that involves yelling, warnings, scaring, and ultimatums is relying on the alarm system to correct behaviour. Parents may need to use alarm techniques when danger is present, but it should be used in moderation. For example, a mother said, "My three-year-old son was going to run across the street to see his father and I couldn't get to him fast enough, so I screamed—'Stop!' He froze and didn't move. I was so thankful he did!"

   The alarm system works best when it isn't overactivated. When adults routinely use alarm methods to "scare kids straight," it can interfere with cultivating strong relationships with them as well as provoke emotional defences. Children are meant to run to parents for help, not run away from them. A father said, "My son smashed into our glass door and broke it. I heard the crash and went to find him, but he had gone to hide. When I found him with his hands bleeding, I asked him why he wouldn't come to me for help. He said he thought he would be in trouble for breaking the door." The father was visibly shaken while considering how his son could have been in danger but did not consult him. It moved the father to consider why his son didn't seek comfort from him and how his son had grown afraid of him.

Parents often use other adults to scare their children, the favourites being police officers, teachers, or principals. When a three-year-old wanted to take her seatbelt off in the stroller, her mother said, "If you don't wear your seatbelt, the police are going to come and take you away from me." When an adult becomes a source of fear, they are displaced from the caretaking role they were meant to serve for a child.

A mother consulted me regarding her five-year-old daughter who was showing symptoms of alarm, including difficulty sleeping, stomachaches, and obsessive behaviour. She said, "When my daughter didn't put on her seatbelt, my husband hit the gas and moved the car and she came out of her car seat and hit her head on the seat in front of her. That was the last time she did this, but I am worried about how my husband disciplines her." If a child faces too much alarm for too long, it can provoke emotional defences to inhibit the vulnerable feelings of alarm, giving rise to symptoms of anxiety and agitation. As a child becomes defended, more alarm will be needed to scare them into better behaviour; in other words, you will need to yell louder or up the ante. One mother said,

> I was visiting my in-laws when my brother's three-year-old son was taking all the books off a bookshelf and throwing them on the

floor. My brother yelled at him to stop, but he seemed oblivious to his threatening voice. As my nephew continued, my brother started yelling louder, until he was screaming at him to stop. The saddest thing was the slow and hesitant reaction of my nephew. He seemed almost unaffected. It made me wonder how many times he had been yelled at like this and what impact this was having on him.

Alarm is meant to move a child to caution, but when adults overuse it, the child will be cautious about trusting adults to care for them. This is especially true for sensitive children, as alarm methods can go quickly over the top and create too much emotional stress, provoking emotional defences.

2. Separation-Based Methods

Separation-based discipline was introduced as an alternative to physical punishment, but the impact on attachment was not considered. Separation-based discipline includes methods such as time-outs, isolation, pretending or threatening to leave a child, withdrawing love, the silent treatment, shunning, and tough love. These measures withdraw the invitation for contact and closeness in order to pressure a child to comply with expectations and requests. Attachment is a child's greatest need; therefore, separation or the threat of it can profoundly affect a child. When the invitation for contact and closeness with a parent is conditional upon performance, it can create a deep sense of insecurity in a child. As a parent said to me, "I was moved when I learned about the insecurity that comes when a child *needs* to be good to keep the attachment. They no longer have the luxury of wanting to be good. They really are placed in a position of keeping the relationship intact as they work at the attachment."

Those who argue for the use of separation-based discipline suggest young children will reflect on their actions when sent away. The capacity to reflect doesn't exist until the 5-to-7 shift. Furthermore, when children are sent away, they are often stirred up with increased frustration and alarm, leaving little room to think about anything else. Time-outs are also viewed as a means of calming a child down and increasing their self-control. The reason some children (not all) appear calm after a time-out is because their alarm system is now pressing down on their emotions so that they can tuck themselves back into relationship with adults. When they emerge from time-outs eager to please and contrite, this is because of attachment alarm.

The threat or use of separation-based methods will increase a child's pursuit for contact and closeness with an adult. They will do just about anything to close the relational gap with their adult, at a cost to their dignity and integrity. This leads to good behaviour, but at what cost to the child or to the relationship? A child care provider conveyed a story of a well-behaved but emotionally troubled child in her care:

> Olivia is so responsible, very giving, polite, and for her young age she acts very mature. I find it a rather sad situation, as she is very alarmed, not spontaneous, even her smiles are forced, and there is not much curiosity. Olivia seems to be opinionated, but she repeats her parent's opinion. I don't know what she thinks, what she believes, what she wants. When Olivia plays with other kids, usually they get hurt. I have watched her push down a girl in a race. Olivia carries a ton of frustration and sadness with her. She suffers from regular tummy aches, but no doctor can find anything wrong. Olivia is paying a high price for being so good! How must she feel, to always be good to hold on to her parents, to feel loved, to live up to their expectations, not to have an invitation to exist otherwise? It must feel dreadful.

A mother spoke to me after a presentation one evening and burst into tears as she said, "I don't know if you noticed, but I was crying as you talked about how children need to feel cared for. Whenever I did anything wrong, my mother would tell me she didn't want me anymore. I was so hurt by this. I tried so hard to be good for her." The heartache in this mother was palpable 30 years later as she stood before me as a mother to two children of her own.

How do we make sense of the children for whom time-outs don't seem to work? Separation-based discipline works only when there is an attachment at stake that a child cares about. If a child is not attached to an adult who uses separation-based discipline, it can increase the likelihood of frustration and attacking behaviour. Sensitive children can find separation very provocative, and it can lead to explosions of behaviour and detaching (see chapter 7).

Separation-based discipline interferes with a child's capacity to rest, play, and grow. When a young child is preoccupied with being good to avoid separation from what they care about, there is less energy left to focus on becoming their own person.

3. Consequences-Based Methods

The use of consequences to control a child's behaviour has become a common discipline technique. Good behaviour is rewarded with privileges, through the use of stickers, charts, or praise. Behaviour that doesn't meet expectations is punished with the removal of possessions, privileges, or activities. One parent asked, "Is it okay to take away my child's favourite stuffed animal they sleep with in order to get them to do things like eat all their food or brush their teeth?" The first question we need to ask is, what is the cost of using what a child cares about against them to achieve compliance?

The use of negative and positive reinforcement as a discipline method stems from behaviour/learning theory and serves to sculpt a child to perform as if mature one incident at a time. It does not consider the instinctive or emotional roots that give rise to troublesome behaviour or the traits of well-behaved children. It uses what a child cares about as leverage, which creates an adversarial relationship. Life does teach through consequences, but this is not what these practices are about. They signal to a child that their dependency on an adult will be exploited whenever compliance is required. As one sensitive four-year-old said to his father, "Dad, you can take that away from me, but I will just decide not to care about anything anymore." It was amazing how this young child could already articulate how his defences would spring into action and inhibit vulnerable feelings when facing separation. Emotional defences can move to protect a child's heart if caring about something sets them up to get hurt. These defences make life easier to bear and children will simply stop caring—about everything.

Educators and parents are increasingly concerned about a lack of caring in kids today, which is also supported by research on empathy.[3] Routine statements such as "I don't care," "It doesn't matter to me," and "Whatever" have become common among our children and youth. In considering where their caring has gone, we have failed to examine discipline methods that use what they care about against them. A father said, "When my kids don't listen, I just take away their screen time and this works every time." A mother told me, "My daughter refuses to be toilet trained, so I get the coldest water to clean her when changing a diaper to teach her a lesson." Another father said, "My son wouldn't sit at the table, he was yelling and screaming, so I told him he couldn't go on an outing with his grandmother." We fail to connect how our children lack caring with how some of our discipline methods do too.

The practice of using consequences to get compliance is a quick fix aimed at changing a child's behaviour immediately. This form of discipline often meets the needs of the adult without considering what is stirring a child up or how to preserve a relationship while steering through incidents. As one parent commented, "It is interesting how behavioural methods of discipline give a parent the illusion of instantly growing a child up, or at least being in control—no wonder these methods are so compelling." Another parent said she became disillusioned with consequences when she realized what was at stake:

> I used to rely on consequences to change behaviour. For example, if my son didn't pick up his toys, he wasn't allowed to come into town with me. Ouch... I didn't realize that I used the threat of separation to "speed" my son up. After presenting "cause and effect" to him, he hurried up, but he was so alarmed that he couldn't think clearly. In fact, it took him longer to get his chore done.

The immature actions of a young child routinely bring consequences that responsible adults must deal with, such as removing toys when they are being thrown at others or moving other kids to safety if a child is lashing out in frustration. There is a difference between using consequences *against* a child and using them *in the service* of being a responsible caretaker. Imposing consequences are what a parent does to change things as a result of a child's behaviour. It is what responsible adults do in the face of a young child's egocentric, impulsive, and inconsiderate actions. It is what we do to compensate for the maturity they are missing. When consequences are used to teach a child a lesson, it only puts them in the lead of behaviour that they are clearly not able to control in the first place. As one mother said, "Being on the computer for very long is not good for my son. He has a big meltdown when asked to come off of it, so I have taken the lead without focusing on his behaviour. I have shortened the amount of time I give him. I expect him not to like it, but I am prepared to help him find his tears." How a child behaves should cue an adult to consider how their child is limited because of immaturity and what they need to do to avoid problems, as a father of a very sensitive boy did after watching his six-year-old play soccer:

> I signed my son up for soccer because he loves it so much. The problem is whenever he gets frustrated on the field, he can't control himself. One day, his team was losing, another child tripped him by accident, and I could see he was mad. He held up his arm and

clotheslined another child. He is not ready to play on a team like this. We have to wait until he has more impulse control because it is too dangerous for other kids out on the field.

Young children can't think twice before acting, which is why consequences routinely fail to alter future performances. Before throwing a toy train, they don't contemplate whether they should use their words instead. They are moved to act and react to the big feelings and instincts inside them. No consequence will ever teach a child what good development is meant to deliver—impulse control. Furthermore, the most difficult behaviour we see from young children is usually a result of being emotionally stirred up and not being in control. Consequences often exacerbate emotions that underlie big problems, as one father explained: "My wife and I were trying to have a conversation about where to go for dinner, but our son kept jumping up between us and wouldn't let us talk. I told him to stop and warned him we wouldn't go out for dinner if he didn't quit it. He wouldn't listen, so I took him up to his room and told him to stay there. He ended up smashing stuff in his room—he just exploded." When a child is stirred up, giving them a consequence can add more fuel to the fire—increasing both frustration and alarm.

Although consequences are problematic when used as a parenting practice, they do serve an important social function. They reinforce the alpha position of the adults in charge and set up expectations that compliance is expected. Schools wouldn't run without principals; someone needs to be seen as being in charge and setting the values and rules for conduct. Consequences allow adults to lead children when there is conflict and satisfy issues around justice or fairness. If adults do not lead in difficult situations, young children will take matters into their own hands. As consequences can create problems in fostering strong adult–child relationships, whenever they are used, they should be depersonalized from the adult and viewed as part of the rules of the overall setting. Adults can also mitigate relational and emotional stress from consequences by bridging and letting a child know a desire for relationship is still present.

Attachment-Safe and Developmentally Friendly Discipline

WHAT IS GOOD discipline? It is the actions of responsible adults who move to deal with the disorder that comes with immaturity. It both protects a child's relationship with their adult and preserves a child's soft heart. Good discipline is what happens before problems arise, when adults work at anticipating issues and get there first. Good discipline arises when an adult aims to understand what is stirring a child up and thinks about how to best address their emotional needs. Good discipline doesn't come from being a perfect parent and often arises out of parental guilt and forming intentions to do things differently next time. Good discipline means not letting a child's behaviour be more important than the relationship. A mother described how her five-year-old was able to convey this to her:

> My daughter came home from kindergarten and started to play with her dolls, giving them a time-out and telling them they were bad. I asked her what was going on and she said the dolls were not listening, so they had to go to a time-out. I asked her how the dolls were feeling about being sent away and she said they were very sad. I asked where she had learned about time-outs given we didn't do them at home and she said, "school." I asked her what we did instead of time-outs and she said, "We just get another chance, Mama."

What young children would really like is some time for maturity to deliver the capacity for self-control so that they can actualize their good intentions. They would also like some support in learning a language of the heart so that they wouldn't have to express their emotions through hits and kicks. They would like time to develop a coherent sense of self so that they wouldn't feel so coerced and have to resist the directions of others.

What every young child would tell us if they could is to please hold on to them, to not take their actions personally, and to love them despite their immaturity. They would tell us they aren't out to make our lives difficult and are only being true to the instincts and emotions inside of them. From a child's perspective, good discipline means an adult still believes in them and knows they will get it right one day. There are many things adults can do to communicate this message to a young child, but this is conveyed most of all as parents generously care for them throughout the most immature period of their life.

Neufeld's Twelve Strategies for Attachment-Safe and Developmentally Friendly Discipline*

THE FOLLOWING TWELVE strategies for attachment-safe and developmentally friendly discipline are meant to help parents lead and assume responsibility for the immature actions of a young child. They are divided into three separate areas: (1) five foundational practices of safe discipline, (2) three discipline strategies that promote healthy development, and (3) four fallback measures for the immature and hard to manage. Following this are special guidelines for handling sibling conflict.

Five Foundational Practices of Safe Discipline

1. DON'T TRY TO MAKE HEADWAY IN THE INCIDENT
When problems arise that evoke strong emotions in a child or adult, it can be better not to try to make headway in the moment. The best

---

* From Gordon Neufeld, "Twelve strategies for attachment-safe and developmentally friendly discipline," *Making Sense of Discipline*, course, Neufeld Institute, Vancouver, BC (011).

bet is to get out of the situation with the relationship intact and address the problem later. This may mean addressing the violation in the moment by dropping the infraction flag, for example, "Hands aren't for hitting, teeth aren't for biting people, and Mommy is not for calling names." You can then bridge the problem behaviour by moving the child along and focusing on something that conveys a desire to still be with them, such as having a snack or reading a story together. You can also let the child know that you will talk to them later about what happened and set a time to deal with the incident. When a child is most stirred up, the focus should be on holding on to the relationship, as this allows a parent to deal with a child when emotions have diminished in intensity.

One of the biggest challenges adults face in managing difficult situations is to do no harm to the relationship and to back off from dealing with a child until they have a better hold on them. Many parents feel compelled to address things head on rather than pull a child closer, the fear being the latter somehow rewards a child or they "get away with it." Dropping the infraction flag signals that something is not okay, and talking to them later ensures problems are addressed. The fear that a child will get away with something is a remnant of a behavioural/learning approach in which children need to be

---

GUIDELINES FOR HANDLING INCIDENTS*

Instead of trying to make headway, aim to do no harm.

1) Address the violation simply (if necessary).
2) Bridge the problem behaviour.
3) Attempt to change or control the situation (NOT the child).
4) Set a date to debrief or address the problem.
5) Exit sooner than later.

* where emotion is involved

Figure 10.2 Taken from Neufeld *Discipline That Doesn't Divide* course

taught to act mature instead of becoming mature through healthy development.

One mother explained how she put these guidelines for handling incidents into practice:

> My three-year-old spilled her milk on the floor on purpose after I told her she couldn't have another cookie. I was so mad, I told her to clean it up and she screamed, "No!" I was so furious, I said, "You will clean that up!" She yelled back at me, "No!" I could feel my frustration escalate to where I wanted to rub her nose in the spilled milk. I got scared by my strong reaction, so I just said, "Everyone out of the kitchen. This isn't working anymore. You will clean up the milk later. We are leaving." I started to walk out and my kids followed me. I ended up in her room, so I started to read to them. My kids came over and sat on my lap, and as I read, I felt the warmth of their bodies and was reminded of how I love to cuddle with them. As my frustration came down, I could engage with my daughter better and told her we needed to go back to the kitchen and we would clean up the milk together. She readily agreed.

2. ENGAGE THE ATTACHMENT INSTINCT BEFORE GOING TO WORK

Young children engage with only one thing or person at a time, so their attachment instincts are not always aimed at the adult who is responsible for them. Collecting a child before telling them what to do helps establish the adult as the one to lead and harnesses the

---

FIVE FOUNDATIONAL PRACTICES OF SAFE DISCIPLINE

1) Don't try to make headway in the incident.
2) Engage the attachment instincts before going to work.
3) Nurture and safeguard the child's desire to be good for you.
4) Know your limits and work within them.
5) Bridge whatever could divide.

Figure 10.3 Taken from Neufeld *Discipline That Doesn't Divide* course

child's motivation to be good. Collecting requires getting their attention in a friendly way, as discussed in chapter 4. Collecting a child is important after any separation, such as sleeping, being away at preschool, or playing on their own. Preschools use circle time to collect young children and determine who is following along and who needs some attention in order to attend better.

Collecting a child before giving them direction seems simple but is easily missed in the hurried pace of family life. Parents are frustrated when young children don't come when called, like at dinnertime, time to leave in the morning, or the start of the bedtime routine. Collecting a child before directing them, especially when cooperation is required, is an effective way to avoid the frustration and resistance that comes when young children feel pushed and not attached to their adults in the moment.

While I was at an indoor play park with my children, a friend asked me for advice on how to get her child to leave. Her three-year-old was having a lot of fun and had disappeared into the tunnels, nets, and slides. I suggested she would need to find her son and collect him before telling him it was time to go. She looked at me in disbelief and said, "Really? That's the best you've got?" I asked her to give it a try and she disappeared into the nets and ladders. She was gone for five minutes until I saw her pop out of one of the slides with her son following behind her. He was looking up at her and taking her cues well. She took him to get his jacket and shoes and without a word waved goodbye and was out the door. She told me later that leaving the park and other events had become a lot easier now that she collected her son first.

3. NURTURE AND SAFEGUARD THE CHILD'S DESIRE TO BE GOOD FOR YOU

Many of the popular discipline practices convey mistrust in a child's intentions and a belief children do not naturally want to be good for their adults. Punishment is given to change a child's mind instead of considering how their emotions and impulses got the better of them and eclipsed their good intentions. If a child sees that a parent believes they are trying to do the right thing but made a mistake, it will not only protect the relationship but also preserve the child's willingness to keep aiming in the right direction. This conveys faith in a child they can get it right, tells them they will be loved despite mistakes, and protects everyone's dignity in the process. As one parent said, "It felt like a miracle the first time I noticed my child wanted to be good for me. Discipline became simple and easy and in fact barely needed."

4. KNOW YOUR LIMITS AND WORK WITHIN THEM

Part of dealing with a young child's behaviour is to know when you are at your limit and there is little caring to temper your strong reactions. When a parent loses their own mixed feelings, frustration won't be as tempered by caring and the result is less patience and self-control. When this happens, the challenge for a parent is to find a way to do no harm. A parent asked me, "I get that warmth and attachment are important to kids, but sometimes I just don't feel that way. I am mad, frustrated, tired, and have had enough. What am I supposed to do then?" I replied that caring for a child when we feel least inclined to connect with them means realizing you are at your limit and avoiding actively parenting at that moment. It is about finding a way to take care of yourself and avoiding saying or doing things that would wound a child or create more separation between you.

Parents often ask, "What if I need a time-out so I don't lose it on my kid?" The key is to find a way to take a break without conveying to a child that they are too much to handle. Telling a child you need to get away from them only stirs up their frustration and alarm. However, telling them you have to do laundry, go to the bathroom, or make a cup of tea, or that you will be right back, doesn't convey to the child that they are a source of emotional distress and you have lost your desire to connect with them. When you are at your limit, the responsible thing is to recognize it, protect children from it, and find a way to be the parent they need once again.

5. BRIDGE WHATEVER COULD DIVIDE

Bridging is an attachment ritual that helps convey that there is still a desire for closeness when stormy behaviour arises and actions must be addressed. For example, when a child hits, yells, or lashes out, a parent cannot condone these actions, but they can convey that an invitation for connection still exists despite the infraction. In other words, parents can be firm on behaviour but easy on the relationship. For example, George was upset that his mother wouldn't let him stay at the park. He pleaded, wailed, and went to strike her. She hung on to the relationship and stated, "Mommies aren't for hitting" and "I know you are frustrated and want to stay." As he screamed, she said, "I know you are upset," and started to slowly walk with him towards her car. As she loaded him into the car, she said, "I am looking forward to playing trains with you when we get home." He screamed at her, "I don't want to play with you," to which she replied, "I know you are upset about leaving the park. We will play later."

The act of bridging problem behaviour also conveys to a child that nothing is wrong with them—they aren't too mean, too bad, too upsetting, or too overwhelming for a parent. A child's shortcomings do not become a source of shame or disconnection. Their failures do not set them up for losing a parent's belief that they are lovable just as they are. Bridging is also an effective way to ensure that a child doesn't feel they are too much for a parent to handle. When they see that a parent still wants to be with them, it creates faith that the relationship is strong enough to handle who they are. It creates trust in a parent to steer them through tough situations and towards civilized forms of relating.

Sensitive children are more prone to big emotional reactions when confronted with their problem behaviour. It is helpful to give them space while conveying a desire to help them so as to reduce the intensity of their upset. Debriefing of incidents is probably best done after giving things time to settle, even 24 hours for big incidents. George's mother could have acknowledged later on that he was frustrated at leaving the park and seemed to be having a good time there. She could also solicit some good intentions on his part as to how she wanted him to leave the park next time.

Three Discipline Strategies That Promote Healthy Development

1. SOLICIT GOOD INTENTIONS

Soliciting good intentions is a discipline strategy aimed at getting a child onside and pointing them towards behaving in a certain way. It is a wonderful substitution for consequences, which are focused on extinguishing behaviour *after* it happens. Soliciting a child's intentions happens *before* there are problems and enlists a child's cooperation when their desire to please is highest. As one parent said, "Whenever I take my kids on an outing, I always solicit their good intentions to stay close to me and hold my hand. I can remember a time when I didn't do this and they were having a fit and screaming "no" in the foyer at the science centre. I never forget now to remind

---

THREE DISCIPLINE STRATEGIES THAT PROMOTE HEALTHY DEVELOPMENT

1) SOLICIT GOOD INTENTIONS
Get the child to aim in the right direction.

2) DRAW OUT MIXED FEELINGS
Help the child find the tempering elements that would answer the troubling impulses.

2) COLLECT THE TEARS OF FUTILITY
Help the child find the sadness and disappointment that should come in the wake of encounters with futility.

Figure 10.4 Adapted from Neufeld *Discipline That Doesn't Divide* course

them of the rules when we go on an outing and to get their agreement first. It works like magic."

Soliciting a child's good intentions should work if there is a sufficiently strong relationship between an adult and child between the ages of 2 and 3. A child must be attaching via belonging and loyalty for this strategy to work. If a child is not attached, this strategy could make them want to do the opposite of what is asked because of counterwill. To harness their good intentions, a parent will need to be able to collect the child first. For example, a mother explained,

> My kids started calling their grandmother, "Granny with the short legs" to separate her from their other grandmother. When she heard this name, she was upset and said she didn't want to be referred to by her height. I asked my kids to come up with another name and they said, "Granny with the bad thumb." I told them it couldn't be a body part that didn't work so they said "Granny with the brown hair." When their grandmother came for a visit I solicited a lot of good intentions from them to call her by her new name and they said they would try really hard. When she arrived, they were right on cue and their grandmother was happy with the name change.

Soliciting good intentions is a powerful discipline strategy that helps a child recognize they are meant to eventually direct their own behaviour. It helps a child grasp the steering wheel for their own life and see there are choices they can make. Of course, young children's impulses and emotions will get the better of their intentions at times. For this reason, it is important to come alongside their intention—"You were really trying hard to listen"—rather than focusing on whether they were successful in actualizing it.

2. DRAW OUT MIXED FEELINGS

A young child is unable to mix feelings and thoughts, as discussed in chapter 2, giving rise to impulsive, egocentric, and inconsiderate actions. If development is unfolding well, a child may start to show signs of being able to mix thoughts and feelings between ages 4 and 5, giving rise to a powerful discipline strategy. A parent can try to get this mixing to work outside of incidents when they are debriefing a child. For example, a parent had been through a number of trying nights with her daughter, who refused to brush her teeth. As the mother sidestepped the battles and found ways to reduce the resistance, she started to work on getting her daughter to feel mixed about taking care of her teeth. While talking at bedtime, the mother said, "One part of you does not like brushing your teeth at all." Samantha, age 5, said, "I don't like it. Toothpaste is yucky." The mother said she understood, "but I bet there is another side of you that doesn't want to get cavities from the sugar bugs." Her daughter was quiet, so the mother moved on to talk about something else. A few days later, Samantha was yelling that she didn't want to brush her teeth, so her mother promised to come and help her in a minute. When she arrived, Samantha was furiously scrubbing her teeth with her toothbrush. Her mother was surprised and asked, "Why are you brushing your teeth when you didn't want to?" Frothing at the mouth, Samantha yelled, "Because I don't want to get cavities!" When a child starts to experience internal conflict, a whole new level of mature behaviour follows.

It is helpful to draw out mixed feelings after incidents and to allow the child enough distance from an event so that they are not hijacked by strong emotion. The goal in drawing out the tempering element is to put the child in the middle of conflicting feelings and thoughts so as to eventually sandwich them together.

A father relayed the following conversation that happened while debriefing his daughter after a fight with her younger brother:

Father: "Your brother gave you a really big scratch on your face today. I know you were really frustrated with him. Why do you think he was so frustrated with you?"

Katie: "I told him I didn't want to play trains with him, so he scratched me."

Father: "He loves his trains, he must have been upset. You got hurt too. It's hard to have a little brother sometimes, isn't it?"

Katie: "Yeah, my brother can be mean."

Father: "Is there a side of you that still likes to play with him and feels sorry for what you said?"

Katie: "Yeah, I still like playing with him and I am sorry too."

When drawing out the mixed feelings, it is important to collect the child and be in a position of influence. A child's memory of an event can be used to bring back their experience and create the internal conflict between their thoughts and feelings. The more a parent normalizes and makes room for inner conflict, the more experience a child will have in using this to temper their strong feelings as they arise. Working outside of the incidents will translate into better self-control in the heat of the moment.

3. COLLECT THE TEARS OF FUTILITY

There are times when a young child is up against the things they cannot change, such as not getting to stay up late, not being able to have another cookie, or having to share toys. Instead of imposing consequences, applying sanctions, or alarming a child, a parent can simply say no, offer comfort, and collect the tears of futility, as discussed in chapter 7. There are times when the best discipline strategy is to present what won't work, can't work, and shouldn't work.

As a child becomes more willful, their encounters with futility and the need to collect their tears will probably increase. For example, a mother relayed the following story about her two-year-old child:

We were at the beach and I put a sun hat on my daughter, but she kept taking it off despite trying to distract her. I put it back on her head and said, "No, we need to wear our hat." She looked at me and tore it off again. I said, "No" and put it back on her head. This went on for about 20 minutes and she cried and screamed. I was patient with her, telling her I understood she was frustrated, but decided this was a good time for me to collect her tears about a hat that needed to be worn."

These small encounters with futility are helpful in setting the stage for the bigger issues that will come.

Four Fallback Measures for the Immature

1. ASSUME RESPONSIBILITY FOR THE CHILD WHO GETS IN TROUBLE
When a child is consistently getting into trouble, the best discipline strategy is to put them under the watchful eye of an adult who assumes responsibility for guiding their interactions and dealing with their behaviour before it becomes a problem. For example, putting kids around a sand table with a child who is full of attacking energy only sets someone up to get hurt. If adults know there will probably be a fight, then supervision is required to help the children share and take turns.

If a child doesn't move to caution and displays little fear, it is only adult supervision that helps them stay out of harm's way. If they fight consistently with their sibling or other children, then they can't be left alone. Adults need to compensate for a child, particularly one who is easily emotionally stirred up and struggling. If a child is unpredictable to be around, then an adult needs to be in charge of keeping people safe and protecting the child's dignity.

FOUR FALL-BACK MEASURES FOR THE IMMATURE

1) **ASSUME RESPONSIBILITY** for the child who gets into trouble.
2) **USE STRUCTURE AND RITUAL** to orchestrate chaotic behaviour.
3) **CHANGE THE CIRCUMSTANCES** that control the child.
4) **SCRIPT** the behaviour of the immature.

Figure 10.5 Taken from Neufeld *Discipline That Doesn't Divide* course

2. USE STRUCTURE AND ROUTINE TO ORCHESTRATE
CHAOTIC BEHAVIOUR

Young children are prone to counterwill reactions, so structure and routine can help orchestrate their interactions at times when they are most prone to be resistant, such as when facing bedtimes, meals, and hygiene tasks. When a child adjusts to structure and routine, fewer demands and commands will need to be made to ensure compliance. Structure and routine also help a young child orient and anticipate what will happen each day, making transitions easier and less upsetting.

3. CHANGE THE CIRCUMSTANCES THAT CONTROL THE CHILD

An adult cannot control a child who is not in control of themselves, though this doesn't stop many adults from trying. When a child is really stirred up, it is often better to change the circumstances in order to change their behaviour. For example, change the scenery or distract a child, by heading outside or going to play something they like. One father said, "Whenever my sensitive son is tired and grumpy, he is unmanageable. Whenever he starts to go loopy on me, I just try to find something different to do, like read a cookbook to decide on a dessert, play some music, watch a funny video on the computer about animals, or just get him outside."

4. SCRIPT THE BEHAVIOUR OF THE IMMATURE

Young children can't read context well, so they are often unaware how to conduct themselves appropriately in certain situations. Adults can give a child a script for their behaviour, including step-by-step instructions on how to act. There are many types of interactions and behaviours that can be scripted, including manners and dealing with peer conflict. For example, a mother of a four- and a two-year-old said,

> My children went to my in-laws for a visit and when they returned,
> my mother-in-law said they had been mean to her dog. My kids

have never been around a dog, so they didn't have a clue what to do with one. I told them the dog was afraid of them and they needed to treat it differently. I asked them what they thought they could do to be nicer. My eldest said, "We won't put stickers on it. We won't colour it with markers. We won't ride it." Once I agreed these were all good ideas, I got one of their stuffed animals and taught them how to pet and be gentle with a dog. The next visit with the dog went much better.

Special Guidelines for Handling Sibling Conflict

WHEN SIBLINGS OR young children fight, adults need to assume responsibility for restoring order. There are several principles to bear in mind when dealing with sibling conflict:

- *Assume the lead in guiding interactions.* Young children shouldn't be left to sort out their own conflicts. Given that they lack consideration and the ability to think about both sides of the story simultaneously, they are unlikely to come up with a fair or civilized resolution to their disputes. The adult needs to communicate that they are in charge and will decide how to find a way through the impasse.

- *Don't play judge and jury.* When an adult takes up a position as a judge and jury and delivers a verdict on sibling conflict, a young child will see it as a breach of the relationship if the adult does not side with them. Furthermore, if a parent does not witness the conflict, they have to rely on incomplete information and perspectives that lack an appreciation of context, making unfair judgements possible.

- *Come alongside each child's experience.* Although an adult cannot agree with how children have responded to each other, they *can* come alongside each one's feelings: "I see you are upset your sister doesn't want to play with you" and "I see you are upset that your brother keeps following you around and wants to play." Coming alongside each child's feelings will help preserve the relationship and convey that someone is in charge. It can be done in private with each child or in the middle of disagreements, as a parent feels is appropriate.

- *Don't request that sorrys be delivered unless they are genuinely felt.* Instead of demanding that children say sorry to each other, request that they apologize when they have sorrys in them. A child may need a prompt later: "Now might be a good time to say sorry if you feel this way." Detaching their sorry from any remorse, however, will do more harm than good.

- *Look for underlying reasons when conflict is chronic and pervasive.* When a young child is full of attacking energy, it is important to consider why they are experiencing so much frustration. Sometimes they experience too much separation and their frustration is released on the most available subject—siblings. Sometimes a child is missing their caring feelings and they are full of alarm or attacking energy. The restoration of vulnerable feelings will reduce sibling conflict.

What adults need to bear in mind most of all as they discipline young children is that children know much better than they behave. They have desires to be good for those they are attached to, but their immaturity gets in the way. Discipline that is contrived and that uses attachment alarm to change their behaviour courts disaster— it erodes the conditions needed to foster growth and maturity. We cannot lead a child whose heart we do not have. Good discipline preserves right relationships with adults and the soft hearts of young children.

How Young Children
Grow Adults Up

Tell me whom you love and I will tell you who you are.
ARSÈNE HOUSSAYE[1]

ANNA FELT UTTERLY defeated and pleaded with people around her, "Is there anything else you can do for me?" The previous ten hours of her life had filled her body with pain, her heart with anticipation, and her mind with self-doubt.

At midnight, her body had decided it was time. As her husband started counting contractions, she told him he needed to pack her bag from her to-pack list. While Gregg counted seconds, his attention divided between his watch and Anna, he read her writing: "Pack relaxed and comfortable clothes." With the weight of responsibility on his shoulders to get things right, he proceeded to hold up pants and tops for approval. He was met with Anna's ferocious cries of "Seriously? Does that look relaxing to you?" And so in the early hours of the morning, Anna and Gregg began their journey towards parenthood—unsure, determined, excited, overwhelmed, and eagerly awaiting the child they had already started to love.

As the sun came up, Anna's mother and her doula arrived to escort them to the hospital. After seven hours of labour her contractions were a minute and a half apart; Anna had ten of them on her way to the car. She remembers feeling furious that people wouldn't get out of the way on the road. "I was looking at the clock—6:52—these people are going to work? The whole world is acting normal, like this is just like every other day? Couldn't they see I was in labour? I wanted to bellow like Fezzik from *The Princess Bride*—EVERYBODY MOVE—and just get to the hospital."

At the hospital, her pleading for pain relief led to being given gas. "I became so attached to the gas, it became my ritual of breathing. I had to take such deep breaths with Gregg helping me." After two and a half hours, she was told the labour wasn't progressing. She was stuck in the perpetual motion of pain and exasperation. For the first time since labour had begun, Anna felt defeated, like she had no control over things—"It was just happening to me."

Anna remembers clearly the moment things began to change. Her doula looked at her squarely and said, "You are doing this." Anna says, "For whatever reason it triggered this feeling I could do this, that I was doing everything I needed to be doing." The labour shifted almost immediately. In the middle of the intense pain, Anna remembers feeling like an active participant in the labour again. It was like "my body answered and it started doing things on a more intuitive basis and being less reactive." In hindsight she says the hardest thing was having to be this "mature person and not panic, and realize the more you fight, the harder it was on you. I needed to release myself to this place and pain in order to find my way through." For the next two hours, with every breath, Anna focused on a few words to guide her. She began to talk to her son and repeat to him over and over again, "I invite you, I invite you, I invite you." It was upon this generous invitation to exist that her son, Matthew, came into the world.

As I listened to Anna's story, I was moved to consider all that comes with parenthood—the life-altering and transformational experience that it is. There is pain, work, exasperation, frustration, worry, agony, defeat, overwhelm, and anticipation that never seems to end. But there is also the ignition of deep instincts and emotions that thrust, fuel, and steer a parent towards discovering that they are the answer to their child. Regardless of how we claim our children—through adoption, C-section, surrogacy, or vaginal birth—the activation of these instincts and emotions is how young children grow their parents up. We may not have wanted a growth experience, a road map to our imperfections, or a spotlight on our immaturity, but this is what comes with raising a child. As we move to assume the weight of responsibility for taking care of them, we are delivered into parenthood. Being a parent is more than just a list of things we do; it is about who we are to our children and who we become because of loving them.

The Emotions That Come with Parenthood

PARENTS HAVE FEELINGS too—lots of them. Sometimes these are unexpected, unwanted, and troublesome, but they will happen to us nonetheless. Sometimes we may even find, to our dismay, that we can also have temper tantrums and get stuck in resistance just like our child. Raising a child represents a unique opportunity for emotional maturation, but it won't happen without some growing pains. Children can draw emotions out of us that we didn't even know we struggled with. Like mirrors for our immaturities, they reveal our weakest places and introduce us to ourselves all over again. Do we like what we see? Are we disturbed by the image of ourselves as we look at our children hurt, confused, or scared? Many parents ask whether there is a way to get rid of all the emotions that flood, overwhelm, and tumble out on top of their young child. The answer is no, but it doesn't mean we can't take responsibility for our emotional responses.

Emotional maturity doesn't mean a parent is no longer stirred up by their feelings in relation to their child. Emotional maturity is how we accept and make room for the feelings our children raise in us. As parents we can form intentions of how we want to handle our own heart's contents. In doing so, we will likely find that a young child's immature reactions push us towards becoming more tempered in our reactions. For example, a parent's frustration is met with caring to create self-control, and fear is met with desire to form courage. Perhaps the greatest virtue we can aspire to is to be a tempered human being. There is no other force like that of a young child to test our limits. Caring for them will call forth the need for self-control, patience, consideration, courage, forgiveness, and sacrifice— the six virtues of a mature temperament discussed in chapter 2. It is one of life's paradoxes that as we grow our young children up, they give rise to the same process inside us. The synchronicity of growth in a parent and child is ironic if not beautiful. To ensure that this growth occurs, we cannot let our love for our children grow cold. We need enough contact and closeness so that we can fulfill our parent role. We cannot outsource being our child's answer to anyone else.

As a parent takes responsibility for their emotions, they should seek to preserve their relationship with their child and shield their child's heart from wounding. They will start to see that the hardest emotions to contend with in their child are the same ones they have not invited in themselves. Sometimes it will be the frustration and tantrums that send a parent spinning. Does a parent struggle to find their own tears when up against the futilities of life? If a parent cannot tolerate their child's constant neediness or dependency, do they struggle with the vulnerable emotions in being an alpha parent and assuming responsibility for another person?

When we come up short in accepting our child's emotions, the answer is not to lose ourselves in self-absorption but to return to our role as a parent. It will be our love for a child that thrusts us towards making sense of what we do with our emotions in the face of theirs. The growing edge of parenthood is when we sit in the middle of the conflict between how we treat a child and how we really want to take care of them. Parents grow more emotionally mature not in isolation but in yearning to be the answer to their child's needs. It is our love for a child that has the power to change us for the better. This requires the courage to look at the distance between how we act and who we want to be for them, and accepting the guilt that will come and letting it steer us in the right direction. The irony is that the more emotionally mature we become, the more we will see all the ways in which we fall short.

There may be times when we need to remove ourselves from active parent duty and give ourselves a break to gather our thoughts and feelings. In doing so, we don't want to convey to a child that we can't handle them, that they are too much for us, or that our feelings have gotten the better of us. We need to proceed only when our frustration can be tempered by our desire to do no harm. There may also be times we need to repair our relationship with a child because our emotions exploded out onto them. As we give them a dignified apology, we don't need to ask if they forgive us, and we shouldn't ask them to relinquish their upset until they are ready.

What Do We Do with Guilt?

WE CANNOT ESCAPE feelings of guilt—this terrain should be well travelled throughout parenthood. Guilt comes in the wake of assuming responsibility for a child and caring for them. This feeling will happen to us, sometimes out of the blue, when bad things occur or something doesn't work, or when we have fallen short in providing for them. Sometimes guilt hides just under the surface of conscious awareness while we try to push it away by directing energy into controlling other things. Our guilt can drive us to overfunction, to become overcautious, or to be overly concerned about a child and their behaviour. Instead of looking at guilt head on, our busyness provides a shield and temporary relief.

Guilt can feel unbearable as we consider our imperfections and inadequacies. However, feelings of guilt are meant to point parents towards what they can change and where they can make a difference, and to help them form intentions to act differently. Yet there are times when the only answer to guilt will be tears. It will be grief that provides rest from the things we regret, the ways we fall short, and how we are powerless to change a child's world like we want to. It is the expression of our guilt through words that frees the tears that need to come. It is our tears that give us reprieve from the gnawing feeling that we aren't good enough parents.

It isn't our children's job to bear parental guilt or hear our sorrow and humility. It isn't our children's job to listen to our unprocessed feelings or how we feel about being their parent. Children aren't meant to see when we feel unsure or lost about what we are doing. Our internal conflict and confusion should be hidden so that they don't feel we can't take care of them. This doesn't mean we can't seek help from other adults when we are stuck. It means that we convey to our children that we are responsible for our own feelings and actions.

Guilt is meant to help a parent get up each day resolved to be their child's answer and to aim towards their caretaking intentions. Its very existence is the expression of our deepest yearning to be a child's best bet.

Becoming the Answer Our Child Needs

THE IMPETUS FOR growth in parenthood comes from accepting responsibility to become the *answer* to a child. This means we seek to be the answer to their hunger for contact and closeness, for sameness, a sense of belonging, significance, love, and being known. It means assuming one's rightful place in leading them and becoming their compass point, comforter, guide, teacher, protector, agent of futility, and home base. At the core, being a child's answer is making sure they feel an invitation to be in our presence across circumstances and conduct. Children shouldn't have to perform to be loved; they should be loved regardless of how they perform.

If there is one thing that matters most in raising a child, it is to strive to become a gracious parent. This requires not making our invitation for relationship conditional upon whether a child measures up to our values. It means that when they fail to please us or don't meet expectations, we still convey a desire to be close. Being a gracious parent is what it means to unconditionally love a child—it is how we become their place of rest so that they can play and grow.

I remember how wonderful it felt as I experienced an unconditional invitation to exist with my grandfather when I was five years old. I was in his garden and wanted to please him, so I worked hard to pick all the flowers and small vegetables off his plants. I folded the ends of my shirt up and made an impromptu bucket to carry the treasure to him. I found him talking to my parents and interrupted them, proudly displaying the contents of his garden in my shirt. I was astonished to see the look of horror on his face. In his wonderful Cockney accent he exclaimed, "Oh, my word! She picked me clean! She picked everything—I won't have vegetables for weeks!" I didn't understand what I had done, but I knew it was wrong. The delight, warmth, and invitation I had longed to gain were replaced with disappointment and upset. I started to back away to find a place to hide in anguish. Then I heard him laugh. It wasn't just a simple laugh but a deep, gut-roaring, nose-snorting laugh. He came to me, gathered me in his arms, and told me it was okay—we were okay. I saw the twinkle in his eyes return and my heart started to beat slowly once more. I vowed never to pick his vegetables without asking. What he conveyed was that there was nothing I could do to separate me from his love.

We cannot become our child's answer through books, someone else's mantras, or directions. This place must be born inside us from alpha instincts and vulnerable emotions. It is as much about caring as it is responsibility. When we look to the external world to steer us in being a parent, we do not listen to our own hearts and minds. When we believe instructions are necessary to be a child's best bet, we will feel shame when we lack answers instead of feeling we *are* a child's answer. When we don't use our insight and intuition to make sense of a child, we will believe that someone else's answers are superior to our own.

As we endeavour to become a child's best bet, perhaps they are also ours. Their immaturity calls forth our maturity. Their intense need for relationship forces us to live in communion with others to help raise them. They remind us daily of the mystery, splendour, and roots from which we unfold as humans. Some say Nature is mad in delivering us such immature beings, yet I cannot help but think her wise. As adults, we face forward into aging and separation, but in holding on to our children, we are forced to look back to our beginnings. Nature ties the ends of our life cycle together, the old connected to the new, the endings fused to the beginnings, opposites entwined, the paradoxical rendered seamless, endless. These invisible ties of relationships hold us together—the human life cycle unfolding generation after generation.

What Does It Mean to Rest, Play, Grow?

PROVIDING REST IS the most significant contribution parents can make to help a young child reach their full human potential. Parents must labour in matters of love and caretaking so that a child does not. Parents will need to assume responsibility in conveying that they are the answer to a child's hunger for relationship. They will need to provide for and protect the conditions that allow a child to play, thrive, and flourish. They will need to trust that they are a good enough parent despite guilt, imperfections, and inadequacies.

When we bring a child to rest in our care, they are free to grow into the people that only our love can make them. In return, we are transformed into the parents that only our love for a child can make us. We will need to bear the sacrifices that are required, endure the tests of patience and loyalty that will come, tolerate the flaws in ourselves that will appear in the wake of trying to be their answer, and have courage to believe we are their best bet. Parenthood has never been about perfection but about freeing our children from working for love and allowing them to take our invitation for relationship for granted.

The goal in parenting is to gradually retire to a consulting role as we watch a child become their own person and take the steering wheel in their own life. As we face old age, we can take comfort in knowing we were the gardeners they needed. After retiring from work, my father told me he woke up one morning feeling a sense of gratitude that he had lived long enough to know both his grandparents and his grandchildren. He brought to mind that not only do we rest as a child in the care of others, we also find rest as adults in being a caretaker for others.

The early years are magical ones, but we are in danger of losing the beauty and innocence of this age—the magic young children believe in, their integrity, and the purity of living one emotion and thought at a time. Early childhood is a special time full of impulsive and egocentric behaviour that will bring both joy and frustration. The young have a right to their immaturity, and our energies would be well spent in considering how to let them be young while keeping them safe, letting them play, providing limits, and fostering the relational gardens for them to grow in.

In the process of writing Rest, Play, Grow, I asked my children if they felt they were special and loved by their father and me. Their answer has changed from when they were young children, especially as they enter their adolescent years. Instead of telling me they "don't know why they are loved and special," they told me, "because I am yours and because I am me." In their few words they have managed to capture the essence of what it means to rest, play, and grow—because I am at home with you, I am free to grow into me. My children remind me daily that although we are born in an immature form, we unfold in our capacity to be fully human one moment at a time.

About the Neufeld Institute

THE NEUFELD INSTITUTE is committed to putting parents back into the driver's seat with regard to their own children. Our mission is to use developmental science to rejoin parents and teachers to their own natural intuition. All our endeavours are based on the understanding that the context for raising children is their attachment to those responsible for them.

The Neufeld Institute is headquartered in Vancouver, Canada, and uses the latest Internet technology to provide training and education throughout the world. Neufeld faculty and Neufeld course facilitators are currently practising in ten countries: Canada, the United States, Mexico, Germany, Israel, Finland, Sweden, Denmark, Australia, and New Zealand.

The Neufeld Institute offers an insight-based parent education program through online and onsite courses and presentations as well as a continuing education program for parents, educators, and professionals. Training programs exist for those wishing to facilitate Neufeld Institute courses as well as for helping professionals seeking to practise this approach through parent consulting.

Our online campus supports the growing number of those who are teaching and practising the paradigm throughout the world. This campus is accessible to individuals in five languages and serves to join the sparks that are happening in diverse settings around the globe.

The Neufeld Institute is incorporated as a not-for-profit society in British Columbia and registered as a charitable organization in Canada. Please see our website for more information.

About Dr. Gordon Neufeld

THE FOUNDER OF the Neufeld Institute is a Vancouver-based developmental psychologist with 40 years of experience with children and youth and those responsible for them. A foremost authority on child development, Dr. Neufeld is an international speaker, a best-selling author (*Hold On to Your Kids*), and a leading interpreter of the developmental paradigm. Dr. Neufeld has a widespread reputation for making sense of complex problems and for opening doors for change. Formerly involved in university teaching and private practice, he now devotes his time to teaching and training others, including educators and helping professionals, through the Neufeld Institute. He has developed a series of courses for parents, teachers, and professionals. Dr. Neufeld appears regularly on radio and television. He is a father of five and a grandfather of six.

Neufeld Materials

THE THEORETICAL MATERIAL and images in *Rest, Play, Grow* are taken or adapted from the following courses and presentation with the generous permission of Gordon Neufeld.

COURSES
- *Neufeld Intensive I: Making Sense of Kids*
- *Neufeld Intensive II: The Separation Complex*
- *Making Sense of Preschoolers*
- *Making Sense of Play*
- *The Attachment Puzzle*
- *Alpha Children*

- *Heart Matters: The Science of Emotion*
- *Making Sense of Aggression*
- *Making Sense of Anxiety*
- *Making Sense of Attention Problems*
- *Making Sense of Counterwill*
- *Discipline That Doesn't Divide*

PRESENTATION

- "What About Me? Reflections on Growing Up as Adults," Keynote Address by Gordon Neufeld, Neufeld Annual Conference 2013, Vancouver, BC

Acknowledgements

IT HAS BEEN both formidable and fulfilling to write a book about young children based on the theoretical work of Dr. Gordon Neufeld. As I endeavoured to provide insight into young children, I was immersed in making sense of book writing, publishing, and storytelling, and of myself as a writer. Without the support of the following people, insight would not have been gleaned nor would a book have been published. I am sincerely grateful and appreciative to those who cared enough about this project to share their time, stories, and expertise with me.

The developmental science in *Rest, Play, Grow* was brought to life by the stories generously shared with me by parents, child care providers, educators, helping professionals, and Neufeld faculty and course facilitators. Although their identities cannot be revealed, they were uniform in their desire to share in the hope their story would help a parent understand their young child better.

Many people were supportive of this project, giving me their time and feedback, reading chapters, sharing ideas, unearthing stories, and encouraging me to continue writing, in particular, Bridgett Miller, Liz Hatherell, Kat Howe, Catherine Kirkness, Sara Easterly, Marie Chernen, Stephanie Gold, Eva Svensson, Bria Shantz, Tamara Strijack, Genevieve Schreier, April Quan, Heather Ferguson, Dagmar Neubronner, Heather Beach, Tracy Berretta, Tania Culham, Linda

Quennec, Diana Teichrieb, Traci MacNamara, and Jennifer MacDonald. Thank you for all of your support; it helped me stay grounded and focused on what parents really want to know.

I wish to thank Traci Costa and all the folks at Peekaboo Beans for their amazing support and for believing in play as much as I do. You make beautiful clothes, are champions of children's play, and make this world a better place for kids to grow up in.

I am thankful to Joy Neufeld for coming up with the phrase "Rest, Play, Grow," which encapsulates the developmental road map with both simplicity and elegance. Gail Carney, a cherished faculty member at the Neufeld Institute, graciously shared her story for the play chapter in the few weeks before her passing, in keeping with her true alpha caretaking nature. My only regret is that I did not get the chance to share this book with her. I am also grateful for the ongoing support of the Neufeld Institute and all of the compassionate and dedicated people there who endeavour to help adults make sense of their kids. Working with you reminds me of a saying I once read: "You can move faster on your own, but farther when you move together." I like being "together" with all of you.

I was fortunate to find a publishing dream team at Page Two Strategies, who worked diligently and professionally to bring *Rest, Play, Grow* to life. Trena White managed the book project and steered it skillfully, and Megan Jones seamlessly matched me with all the right people under tight timelines. Stephanie Fysh, my copyeditor, was meticulous in her care of the manuscript. Nayeli Jimenez used her design skills to create a beautiful book layout and cover as well as recreate images from presentation slides. Shirarose Wilensky, my editor, was thoughtful in her revisions and intuitive with her suggestions, working tirelessly to bring *Rest, Play, Grow* to life with me word by word.

I wish to thank Bridgett Miller, my social media maven, who generously guided me through the online world and introduced me to people she believed were aligned with our message. Her compassion, humour, and strong caring alpha nature made the journey to market a fun adventure.

I would like to express my sincere gratitude to Elana Brief, who generously gave her time to unearth source material and compile all of the references, to read and edit chapters, to provide content suggestions, and to lend both moral support and humour throughout the writing of *Rest, Play, Grow*. The image of you in the library stacks with a preschooler sitting on you as you look for source material still brings a smile to my face.

I am indebted to Gordon Neufeld for generously sharing with me his material, his enthusiasm as a teacher, his brilliance as a theorist, and his warm invitation to learn and work with him, and for encouraging me every step of the way. You are a true champion of all children and the answer for parents who strive to be their child's best bet.

To my parents, sisters, and friends, thank you for your encouragement and understanding as I removed myself from your company to write. I love you all dearly. To Chris, with whom I share the journey of parenthood, and to my children, Hannah and Madeline—you are my place of rest where I continue to play and grow.

About the Author

DR. DEBORAH MACNAMARA is a clinical counsellor and educator with more than 25 years' experience working with children, youth, and adults. She is on faculty at the Neufeld Institute, operates a counselling practice, and speaks regularly about child and adolescent development to parents, child care providers, educators, and mental health professionals. She continues to write, do radio and television interviews, and speak to the needs of children and youth based on developmental science. Deborah resides in Vancouver, Canada, with her husband and two children.

Notes

Introduction: Why Making Sense Matters

1. Jiddu Krishnamurti, *Education and the Significance of Life* (1953; New York: Harper, 1981), p. 47.

Chapter 1: How Adults Grow Young Children Up

1. Thích Nhất Hạnh, *How to Love* (Berkeley, CA: Parallax Press, 2015), p. 10.

2. Michael S. Pritchard, "On taking emotions seriously: A critique of B.F. Skinner," *Journal for the Theory of Social Behaviour* 6 (1976): 211–32.

3. Carl R. Rogers, Howard Kirschenbaum, and Valerie Land Henderson, *Carl Rogers: Dialogues: Conversations with Martin Buber, Paul Tillich, B.F. Skinner, Gregory Bateson, Michael Polanyi, Rollo May, and Others* (Boston: Houghton Mifflin, 1989).

4. John B. Watson, *Behaviorism* (Chicago: University of Chicago Press, 1930), p. 82.

5. Gordon Neufeld and Gabor Maté, *Hold On to Your Kids: Why Parents Need to Matter More Than Peers* (New York: Ballantine Books, 2014); Daniel J. Siegel, *The Developing Mind: How Relationships and the Brain Interact to Shape Who We Are* (New York: Guilford Press, 2012).

6. Jaak Panksepp and Lucy Biven, *The Archaeology of Mind: Neuroevolutionary Origins of Human Emotions* (New York: W.W. Norton, 2012); Antonio Damasio, *Descartes' Error: Emotion, Reason, and the Human Brain* (London: Vintage Books, 2006).

7. Quoted in Larry K. Brendtro, "The vision of Urie Bronfenbrenner: Adults who are crazy about kids," *Reclaiming Children and Youth: The Journal of Strength-Based Interventions* 15 (2006): 162–66, http://www.cyc-net.org/cyc-online/cyconline-nov2010-brendtro.html.

8. Gordon Neufeld, *Neufeld Intensive I: Making Sense of Kids*, course (Neufeld Institute, Vancouver, BC, 2013), http://neufeldinstitute.org/course/neufeld-intensive-i-making-sense-of-kids/; Gordon Neufeld, *Neufeld Intensive II: The Separation Complex*, course (Neufeld Institute, Vancouver, BC, 2007), http://neufeldinstitute.org/course/neufeld-intensive-ii/; Siegel, *The Developing Mind*; Robert Karen, *Becoming Attached: First Relationships and How They Shape Our Capacity to Love* (Oxford: Oxford University Press, 1998); John Bowlby, *Attachment and Loss* (New York: Basic Books, 1969); Sue Gerhardt, *Why Love Matters: How Affection Shapes a Baby's Brain* (London: Brunner-Routledge, 2004); Thomas Lewis, Fari Amini, and Richard Lannon, *A General Theory of Love* (New York: Random House, 2000).

9. John Bowlby, "Maternal care and mental health," *Bulletin of the World Health Organization* (1951).

10. Kim Parker, "Families may differ, but they share common values on parenting," Pew Research Center (18 September 2014), http://pewrsr.ch/XKvyIf.

11. Gordon Neufeld, *Neufeld Intensive I: Making Sense of Kids*, course (Neufeld Institute, Vancouver, BC, 2013), http://neufeldinstitute.org/course/neufeld-intensive-i-making-sense-of-kids/.

12. Sheldon White, "Evidence for a hierarchical arrangement of learning processes," *Advances in Child Development and Behavior* 2 (1965): 187–220.

13. Arnold J. Sameroff and Marshall M. Haith, editors, *The Five to Seven Year Shift: The Age of Reason and Responsibility* (Chicago: University of Chicago Press, 1996).

14. Neufeld and Maté, *Hold On to Your Kids*.

15. T. Berry Brazelton, *To Listen to a Child: Understanding the Normal Problems of Growing Up* (Reading, MA: Addison-Wesley, 1984), p. 56.

16. Edward Zigler and Elizabeth Gilman, "The legacy of Jean Piaget," in Gregory A. Kimble and Michael Wertheimer, eds., *Portraits of Pioneers in Psychology*, vol. 3 (American Psychological Association, 1998), p. 155.

17. David Elkind, *Miseducation: Preschoolers at Risk* (New York: Knopf, 2006).

18. Margaret Mead, *And Keep Your Powder Dry: An Anthropologist Looks at America* (1942; New York: Berghahn Books, 2000).

19. Sherry Turkle, *Alone Together: Why We Expect More from Technology and Less from Each Other* (New York: Basic Books, 2011).

20. Manuel Castells, *The Rise of the Network Society* (Oxford: Wiley-Blackwell, 2010).

21. Walter Isaacson, *Steve Jobs* (New York: Simon & Schuster, 2011), p. 571.

Chapter 2: The Preschooler Personality: Part Beauty, Part Beast

1. Sophocles, *Ajax* (5th century BC), in *The Dramas of Sophocles Rendered in English Verse, Dramatic & Lyric* (London: Forgotten Books, 2013), pp. 58–59.

2. Gordon Neufeld, *Making Sense of Preschoolers*, course (Neufeld Institute, Vancouver, BC, 2013), http://neufeldinstitute.org/course/making-sense-of-preschoolers/.

3. Lise Eliot, *What's Going On in There? How the Brain and Mind Develop in the First Five Years of Life* (New York: Bantam Books, 2000); Alison Gopnik, *The Philosophical Baby: What Children's Minds Tell Us about Truth, Love, and the Meaning of Life* (New York: Farrar, Straus and Giroux, 2009); Daniel J. Siegel, *The Developing Mind: How Relationships and the Brain Interact to Shape Who We Are* (New York: Guilford Press, 1999).

4. Siegel, *The Developing Mind*.

5. Gopnik, *The Philosophical Baby*.

6. Siegel, *The Developing Mind*.

7. Eliot, *What's Going On in There?*; Siegel, *The Developing Mind*.

8. Eliot, *What's Going On in There?*

9. Eliot, *What's Going On in There?*

10. P. Shaw, K. Eckstrand, W. Sharp, J. Blumenthal, J.P. Lerch, D. Greenstein, L. Clasen, A. Evans, J. Giedd, and J.L. Rapoport, "Attention-deficit/hyperactivity disorder is characterized by a delay in cortical maturation," *Proceedings of the National Academy of Sciences of the United States of America* 104 (2007): 19649–54.

11. Daniel J. Siegel and Tina Payne Bryson, *The Whole Brain Child: 12 Revolutionary Strategies to Nurture Your Child's Developing Mind* (New York: Bantam Books, 2012).

12. Sheldon White, "Evidence for a hierarchical arrangement of learning processes," *Advances in Child Development and Behavior* 2 (1965): 187–220.

13. Siegel, *The Developing Mind*.

14. Eliot, *What's Going On in There?*

15. Arnold J. Sameroff and Marshall M. Haith, editors, *The Five to Seven Year Shift: The Age of Reason and Responsibility* (Chicago: University of Chicago Press, 1996).

16. Thomas S. Weisner, "The 5 to 7 Transition as an Ecocultural Project," in Sameroff and Haith, eds., *The Five to Seven Year Shift*, pp. 295–326.

17. Siegel, *The Developing Mind*; Sue Gerhardt, *Why Love Matters: How Affection Shapes a Baby's Brain* (New York: Brunner-Routledge, 2004); Gordon Neufeld and Gabor Maté, *Hold On to Your Kids: Why Parents Need to Matter More Than Peers* (New York: Ballantine Books, 2014); Thomas Lewis, Fari Amini, and Richard Lannon, *A General Theory of Love* (New York: Random House, 2000).

18. W. Thomas Boyce and Bruce J. Ellis, "Biological sensitivity to context: I. An evolutionary–developmental theory of the origins and functions of stress reactivity," *Development and Psychopathology* 17 (2005): 271–301.

19. Boyce and Ellis, "Biological sensitivity to context."

20. David Dobbs, "The science of success," *The Atlantic* (December 2009), http://www.theatlantic.com/magazine/archive/2009/12/the-science-of-success/307761/.

21. Boyce and Ellis, "Biological sensitivity to context."

22. Gordon Neufeld, *Neufeld Intensive I: Making Sense of Kids*, course (Neufeld Institute, Vancouver, BC, 2013), http://neufeldinstitute.org/course/neufeld-intensive-i-making-sense-of-kids/.

23. Angus Deaton and Arthur A. Stone, "Evaluative and hedonic wellbeing among those with and without children at home," *Proceedings of the National Academy of Sciences of the United States of America* 111 (2014): 1328–33.

24. William N. Evans, Melinda S. Morrill, and Stephen T. Parente, "Measuring inappropriate medical diagnosis and treatment in survey data: The case of ADHD among school-age children," *Journal of Health Economics* 29 (2010): 657–73.

25. Chandra S. Sripada, Daniel Kessler, and Mike Angstadt, "Lag in maturation of the brain's intrinsic functional architecture in attention-deficit/hyperactivity disorder," *Proceedings of the National Academy of Sciences of the United States of America* 111 (2014): 14259–64.

26. Carolyn Abraham, "Failing boys: Part 3: Are we medicating a disorder or treating boyhood as a disease?" *The Globe and Mail* (18 October 2010), http://www.theglobeandmail.com/news/national/time-to-lead/part-3-are-we-medicating-a-disorder-or-treating-boyhood-as-a-disease/article4330080/?page=all.

27. Subcommittee on Attention-Deficit/Hyperactivity Disorder, Steering Committee on Quality Improvement and Management, "ADHD: Clinical practice

guideline for the diagnosis, evaluation, and treatment of attention-deficit/hyper-activity disorder in children and adolescents," *Pediatrics* 128 (2011): 1007-22.

28. Eric R. Coon, Ricardo A. Quinonez, Virginia A. Moyer, and Alan R. Schroeder, "Overdiagnosis: How our compulsion for diagnosis may be harming children," *Pediatrics* 134 (2014): 1013-23; Polly Christine Ford-Jones, "Misdiagnosis of attention deficit hyperactivity disorder: 'Normal behaviour' and relative maturity," *Paediatrics & Child Health* 20 (2015): 200-2.

29. Todd E. Elder, "The importance of relative standards in ADHD diagnoses: Evidence based on exact birth dates," *Journal of Health Economics* 29 (2010): 641-56.

Richard Morrow and colleagues at the University of British Columbia in Canada compared the rates of ADHD diagnosis between the youngest children (born within the month *before* the grade entry cut-off) and the eldest children (born within the month *after*) in a sample of over 900,000 children over age 11; they found the youngest boys were 30 percent more likely to receive an ADHD diagnosis than the eldest, and the youngest girls, 70 percent more likely than the eldest (R.L. Morrow, E.J. Garland, J.M. Wright, M. Maclure, S. Taylor, and C.R. Dormuth, "Influence of relative age on diagnosis and treatment of attention-deficit/hyperactivity disorder in children," *Canadian Medical Association Journal* 184 [2012]: 755-62). According to Todd Elder, if a neurodevelopmental disorder is at the root of the ADHD diagnosis, it should not vary in incidence with a child's birthdate (Elder, "The importance of relative standards in ADHD diagnoses"). Furthermore, children diagnosed with ADHD may grow out of their symptoms with three years of development in the prefrontal cortex, according to Shaw and his colleagues (Shaw et al., "Attention-deficit/hyperactivity disorder is characterized by a delay"). Similarly, Gilliam found that the brain structure responsible for connecting the prefrontal lobes in kids diagnosed with ADHD had a delayed pattern of growth; immaturity is a viable explanation, and maturity a possible remedy, when considering attention problems in young children (M. Gilliam, M. Stockman, M. Malek, W. Sharp, D .Greenstein, F. Lalonde, L. Clasen, J. Giedd, J. Rapoport, and P. Shaw, "Developmental trajectories of the corpus callosum in attention-deficit/hyperactivity disorder," *Biological Psychiatry* 69 [2011]: 839-46).

Not only are kindergarteners more at risk of being diagnosed with attention problems, but the American Academy of Pediatrics states, "There is emerging evidence to expand the age range of the recommendations to include preschool-aged children and adolescents" (Subcommittee on Attention-Deficit/Hyperactivity Disorder, "ADHD," p. 2). Given that there are no pathognomonic markers for ADHD and there is a complete reliance on behavioural descriptions to diagnose it, immaturity can be mistaken for a disorder, according to

Ford-Jones; the implications of stimulant medication on growth and "limited information about and experience with the effects of stimulant medication in children between the ages of 4 and 5 years" is cause for concern (Ford-Jones, "Misdiagnosis of attention deficit hyperactivity disorder").

30. William Crain, *Theories of Development: Concepts and Applications*, 5th edition (Upper Saddle River, NJ: Pearson/Prentice Hall, 2005).

Chapter 3: Preserving Play: Defending Childhood in a Digital World

1. Fred Rogers, Commencement Address, Middlebury College, Middlebury, VT, May 2001, http://www.middlebury.edu/newsroom/commencement/2001.

2. BC Art Teachers' Association, "Honouring Gail Carney" (2015), http://bcata.ca/about-us/tribute.

3. David Elkind, "Can we play?" Greater Good Science Center, University of California, Berkeley (2008), http://greatergood.berkeley.edu/article/item/can_we_play.

4. Elkind, "Can we play?"

5. David Elkind, *The Power of Play: Learning What Comes Naturally* (Cambridge, MA: Da Capo Press, 2007); Nancy Carlsson-Paige, *Taking Back Childhood: Helping Your Kids Thrive in a Fast-Paced, Media-Saturated, Violence-Filled World* (New York: Penguin, 2009); Peter Gray, *Free to Learn: Why Unleashing the Instinct to Play Will Make Our Children Happier, More Self-Reliant, and Better Students for Life* (New York: Basic Books, 2013); Beverly Falk, ed., *Defending Childhood: Keeping the Promise of Early Education* (New York: Teachers College Press, 2012).

6. Madeline Levine, *Teach Your Children Well: Parenting for Authentic Success* (New York: Harper Perennial, 2013).

7. Elkind, "Can we play?"; Kenneth R. Ginsburg, American Academy of Pediatrics Committee on Communications, and American Academy of Pediatrics Committee on Psychosocial Aspects of Child and Family Health, "The importance of play in promoting healthy child development and maintaining strong parent–child bonds," *Pediatrics* 119 (2007): 182–91.

8. Marcy Guddemi, Andrea Sambrook, Sallie Wells, Kathleen Fite, Gitta Selva, and Bruce Randel, "Unrealistic kindergarten expectations: Findings from Gesell Institute's Revalidated Developmental Assessment Instrument," *Proceedings from the Annual Conference for Early Childhood Research and Evaluation* (2012), http://www.highscope.org/files/guddemim_proceedings2012.pdf.

9. D.W. Winnicott, *Playing and Reality* (New York: Basic Books, 1971), p. 73.

10. Mark Twain, *The Adventures of Tom Sawyer* (1876; New York: Oxford University Press, 1996).

11. G. Stanley Hall, *Adolescence: Its Psychology and Its Relations to Physiology, Anthropology, Sociology, Sex, Crime, Religion and Education* (New York: D. Appleton, 1904), p. 235.

12. *Piaget's Developmental Theory: An Overview*, feat. David Elkin, videocassette (San Luis Obispo, CA: Davidson Films, 1989).

13. Stuart L. Brown and Christopher C. Vaughan, *Play: How It Shapes the Brain, Opens the Imagination, and Invigorates the Soul* (New York: Avery, 2009); Pam Schiller, "Early brain development research review and update," *Brain Development: Exchange* (November/December 2010): 26–30; Jaak Panksepp and Lucy Biven, *The Archaeology of Mind: Neuroevolutionary Origins of Human Emotions* (New York: W.W. Norton, 2012); Joe L. Frost, "Neuroscience, play, and child development," paper presented at the IPA/USA Triennial National Conference, Longmont, CO, June 18–21, 1998.

14. Brown and Vaughan, *Play*; Frost, "Neuroscience, play, and child development."

15. Campaign for a Commercial Free Childhood, Alliance for Childhood, and Teachers Resisting Unhealthy Children's Entertainment, *Facing the Screen Dilemma: Young Children, Technology and Early Education* (Boston: Campaign for a Commercial-Free Childhood; New York: Alliance for Childhood, 2012).

16. Bruce D. Perry, Lea Hogan, and Sarah J. Marlin, "Curiosity, pleasure and play: A neurodevelopmental perspective," *Haaeyc Advocate* 20 (2000): 9–12.

17. Perry, Hogan, and Marlin, "Curiosity, pleasure and play."

18. Ginsburg et al., "The importance of play."

19. Frost, "Neuroscience, play, and child development."

20. Jaak Panksepp, "Brain emotional systems and qualities of mental life," in Diana Fosha, Daniel J. Siegel, and Marion Fried Solomon, eds., *The Healing Power of Emotion: Affective Neuroscience, Development, and Clinical Practice* (New York: W.W. Norton, 2009), pp. 1–26.

21. Ginsburg et al., "The importance of play."

22. Ginsburg et al., "The importance of play"; Panksepp, "Brain emotional systems"; Peter Gray, "The decline of play and the rise of psychopathology in children and adolescents," *American Journal of Play* 3 (2011): 443–63.

23. Falk, ed., *Defending Childhood.*

24. Sandra L. Hofferth and John F. Sandberg, "Changes in American children's time, 1981–1997," *Advances in Life Course Research* 6 (2001): 193–229.

25. Ginsburg et al., "The importance of play."

26. Campaign for a Commercial Free Childhood et al., *Facing the Screen Dilemma.*

27. American Academy of Pediatrics, "Media and children" (2015), https://www.aap.org/en-us/advocacy-and-policy/aap-health-initiatives/pages/media-and-children.aspx.

28. Campaign for a Commercial Free Childhood et al., *Facing the Screen Dilemma.*

29. Richard Louv, *Last Child in the Woods: Saving Our Children from Nature-Deficit Disorder* (Chapel Hill, NC: Algonquin Books of Chapel Hill, 2005).

30. Elkind, "Can we play?"

31. Joe L. Frost, *A History of Children's Play and Play Environments: Toward a Contemporary Child-Saving Movement* (New York: Routledge, 2009); Participaction, *Position Statement on Active Outdoor Play* (2015), http://www.participaction.com/wp-content/uploads/2015/03/Position-Statement-on-Active-Outdoor-Play-EN-FINAL.pdf.

32. American Academy of Pediatrics, "Babies as young as 6 months using mobile media" (25 April 2015), http://www.aappublications.org/content/early/2015/04/25/aapnews.20150425-3.

33. Nancy Carlsson-Paige, "Media, technology, and commercialism: Countering the threats to young children," in Falk, ed., *Defending Childhood.*

34. Frost, *A History of Children's Play,* p. xviii.

35. Thomas S. Dee and Hans Henrik Sievertsen, "The gift of time? School starting age and mental health," CEPA Working Paper No. 15-08, Stanford Center for Education Policy Analysis, Stanford University, Stanford, CA (October 2015), https://cepa.stanford.edu/sites/default/files/WP15-08.pdf.

36. Gray, *Free to Learn.*

37. National Association for the Education of Young Children, *The Common Core State Standards: Caution and Opportunity for Early Childhood Education* (Washington, DC: National Association for the Education of Young Children, 2012).

38. Professional Association for Childcare and Early Years, "Concern over 'school-

ification'" (9 July 2013), https://www.pacey.org.uk/news-and-views/news/
archive/2013-news/july-2013/concern-over-schoolification/.

39. Sophie Alcock and Maggie Haggerty, "Recent policy developments and the
'schoolification' of early childhood care and education in Aotearoa New Zealand,"
Early Childhood Folio 17, no. 2 (2013): 21–26.

40. Bryndis Gunnarsdottir, "From play to school: Are core values of ECEC in
Iceland being undermined by 'schoolification'?" *International Journal of Early Years
Education* 22 (2014): 242–50; Dorota Lembrér and Tamsin Meaney, "Socialisation
tensions in the Swedish preschool curriculum: The case of mathematics," *Educare*
2 (2014): 82–98.

41. Christine Gross-Loh, "Finnish education chief: We created a school system
based on equality," *The Atlantic* (March 17, 2014), http://www.theatlantic.com/
education/archive/2014/03/finnish-education-chief-we-created-a-school-system-
based-on-equality/284427/.

42. Tim Walker, "The joyful, illiterate kindergartners of Finland," *The Atlantic*
(1 October 2015), http://www.theatlantic.com/education/archive/2015/10/
the-joyful-illiterate-kindergartners-of-finland/408325/.

43. Council of Ministers of Education, Canada (CMEC), "Programme for International Student Assessment (PISA): Overview" (n.d.), http://www.cmec.ca/251/
Programs-and-Initiatives/Assessment/Programme-for-International-Student-
Assessment-(PISA)/Overview/index.html; see also the various documents
available for PISA 2012 results at http://www.cmec.ca/252/Programs-and-Initia-
tives/Assessment/Programme-for-International-Student-Assessment-(PISA)/
PISA-2012/index.html.

44. Mary-Louise Vanderlee, Sandy Youmans, Ray Peters, and Jennifer Eastabrook,
*Final Report: Evaluation of the Implementation of the Ontario Full-Day Early Learning–
Kindergarten Program* ([Toronto]: Ontario Ministry of Education, Fall 2012), http://
www.edu.gov.on.ca/kindergarten/FDELK_ReportFall2012.pdf; Magdalena Janus,
Eric Duku, and Amanda Schell, *The Full-Day Kindergarten Early Learning Program:
Final Report* (Hamilton, ON: McMaster University, Oct. 2012), http://www.edu.
gov.on.ca/kindergarten/ELP_FDKFall2012.pdf.

45. Harris Cooper, Ashley Batts Allen, Erica. A. Patall, and Amy L. Dent, "Effects
of full-day kindergarten on academic achievement and social development,"
Review of Educational Research 80 (2010): 34–70.

46. James Heckman, "Invest in early childhood development: Reduce deficits,
strengthen the economy," The Heckman Equation (2012), http://heckmanequa-

tion.org/content/resource/invest-early-childhood-development-reduce-deficits-strengthen-economy.

47. Christopher Clouder, "The push for early childhood literacy: A view from Europe," Research Institute for Waldorf Education, *Research Bulletin* 8, no. 2 (2003): 46–52; Comptroller and Auditor General, National Audit Office, *Delivering the Free Entitlement to Education for Three- and Four-Year-Olds* (London: The Stationery Office, 2012).

48. Joan Almon, Nancy Carlsson-Paige, and Geralyn B. McLaughlin, *Reading Instruction in Kindergarten: Little to Gain and Much to Lose* (Alliance for Childhood; Defending the Early Years, 2015), https://deyproject.files.wordpress.com/2015/01/readinginkindergarten_online-1.pdf.

49. Clouder, "The push for early childhood literacy."

50. Joan Almon, "Reading at five: Why?" SouthEast Education Network, SEEN *Magazine* (21 August 2013), http://seenmagazine.us/articles/article-detail/articleid/3238/reading-at-five-why.aspx.

51. Elkind, "Can we play?"

52. Quoted in Valerie Strauss, "How 'twisted' early childhood education has become—from a child development expert," *Washington Post* (24 November 2015), https://www.washingtonpost.com/news/answer-sheet/wp/2015/11/24/how-twisted-early-childhood-education-has-become-from-a-child-development-expert/.

Chapter 4: Hungry for Connection: Why Relationships Matter

1. C.S. Lewis, *The Four Loves* (New York: Harcourt, Brace, 1960).

2. T.S. Eliot, "East Coker," *The Four Quartets* (New York: Harcourt, 1943).

3. Gordon Neufeld, *Neufeld Intensive I: Making Sense of Kids*, course (Neufeld Institute, Vancouver, BC, 2013), http://neufeldinstitute.org/course/neufeld-intensive-i-making-sense-of-kids/.

4. Jaak Panksepp and Lucy Biven, *The Archaeology of Mind: Neuroevolutionary Origins of Human Emotions* (New York: W.W. Norton, 2012).

5. Kerstin Uvnäs Moberg, *The Oxytocin Factor: Tapping the Hormone of Calm, Love, and Healing* (Cambridge, MA: Da Capo Press, 2003).

6. Panksepp and Biven, *The Archaeology of Mind*.

7. John Bowlby, *Attachment and Loss* (New York: Basic Books, 1969).

8. Bowlby, *Attachment and Loss*.

9. Dorothy Corkille Briggs, *Your Child's Self-Esteem: The Key to His Life* (Garden City, NJ: Doubleday, 1970), p. 55.

10. Lise Eliot, *What's Going On in There? How the Brain and Mind Develop in the First Five Years of Life* (New York: Bantam Books, 2000).

11. D.W. Winnicott and Claire Winnicott, *Talking to Parents* (Reading, MA: Addison-Wesley, 1993), pp. 58–59.

12. Benjamin Spock, *The Common Sense Book of Baby and Child Care* (New York: Duell, Sloan and Pearce, 1946).

13. Gordon Neufeld and Gabor Maté, *Hold On to Your kids: Why Parents Need to Matter More Than Peers* (New York: Ballantine Books, 2004), pp. 29–30 .

14. Larry K. Brendtro, "The vision of Urie Bronfenbrenner: Adults who are crazy about kids," *Reclaiming Children and Youth: The Journal of Strength-Based Interventions* 15 (2006): 162–66.

15. Gabor and Maté, *Hold On to Your Kids*, p. 264.

Chapter 5: Who's in Charge? The Dance of Attachment

1. William Blake, "The Little Black Boy," *Songs of Innocence* (London, 1789).

2. Gordon Neufeld, *Alpha Children: Reclaiming Our Rightful Place in Their Lives*, course (Neufeld Institute, Vancouver, BC, 2013), http://neufeldinstitute.org/course/alpha-children/.

Chapter 6: Feelings and Hurts: Keeping Children's Hearts Soft

1. Blaise Pascal, *Pascal's Pensées* (New York: E. P. Dutton, 1958), p. 79.

2. Michael S. Pritchard, "On taking emotions seriously: A critique of B.F. Skinner," *Journal for the Theory of Social Behaviour* 6 (1976): 211–32.

3. Jaak Panksepp, "Brain emotional systems and qualities of mental life," in *The Healing Power of Emotion: Affective Neuroscience, Development, and Clinical Practice*, edited by Diana Fosha, Daniel J. Siegel, and Marion Fried Solomon, pp. 1–26 (New York: W.W. Norton, 2009).

4. Antonio R. Damasio, *Descartes' Error: Emotion, Reason, and the Human Brain* (New York: Putnam, 1994).

5. Diana Fosha, Daniel J. Siegel, and Marion Fried Solomon, eds., *The Healing Power of Emotion: Affective Neuroscience, Development, and Clinical Practice* (New York: W.W. Norton, 2009), p. vii.

6. Thomas Lewis, Fari Amini, and Richard Lannon, *A General Theory of Love* (New York: Random House, 2000), p. 64.

7. The concept of emotional defences once postulated by Freud has been revisited due to advances in neuroscience and new understandings of human emotion and consciousness. Neuropsychologist Mark Solms states, "It is possible to find the neurological correlates of some traditional psychoanalytic concepts and thereby to set them on a firm, organic foundation"(Mark Solms and Oliver Turnbull, *The Brain and the Inner World: An Introduction to the Neuroscience of Subjective Experience* [New York: Other Press, 2002], p. 104). V.S. Ramachandran argues we now have the basis to understand how the human mind erects defensive emotional processes (V.S. Ramachandran, D. Rogers-Ramachandran, and S. Cobb, "Touching the phantom limb," *Nature* 377, no. 6549 [12 October 1995]: 489–90, and V.S. Ramanchandran, "Phantom limbs, neglect syndromes, repressed memories and Freudian Psychology," in *International Review of Neurobiology*, vol. 37: *Selectionism and the Brain*, edited by Olaf Sporns and Giulio Tononi [New York: Academic Press, 1994]). In her writing on the neurophysiology of psychology, Kathleen Wheeler provides an overview of the construct of emotional defence as well as neuroscientific evidence on how parts of the emotional brain orchestrate this (*Psychotherapy for the Advanced Practice Psychiatric Nurse* [Maryland Heights, MO: Mosby, 2007]).

Neuroscientific research examining the inhibition of the emotional centres and processes in the brain has been the primary focus of trauma specialists. Bessel Van der Kolk's research on trauma explores the role of the prefrontal cortex in exerting an inhibitory influence over the limbic system and in regulating emotion (Bessel Van der Kolk, Alexander C. McFarlane, and Lars Weisaeth, *Traumatic Stress: The Effects of Overwhelming Experience on Mind, Body, and Society* [New York: Guilford Press, 2006]). Pat Odgen discusses three categories of defences, outlining how they aid in emotional survival, creating feelings of safety as well as impact overall functioning ("Emotion, mindfulness, and movement: Expanding the regulatory boundaries of the window of affect tolerance," in Fosha, Siegel, and Solomon, eds., *The Healing Power of Emotion*). Ad Vingerhoets links emotional distress and trauma with the absence of vulnerable emotions, stating that people "feel numb, emotionally empty and 'detached,' and cannot produce tears. It is as if they are indifferent and do not experience any affection for or do not care about other people even those very close to them" (*Why Only Humans Weep: Unravelling* the Mysteries of Tears [Oxford: Oxford University Press, 2013], p. 177).

Neuroscientists Jaak Panksepp and Antonio Damasio state that unconscious emotional arousal is possible, distinguishing feeling states from emotional ones. Damasio states that there is "no evidence that we are conscious of all of our feelings, and much to suggest that we are not" (The Feeling of What Happens: Body and Emotion in the Making of Consciousness [New York: Houghton Mifflin Harcourt, 2009], p. 36; for Panksepp, see Jaak Panksepp and Lucy Biven, The Archaeology of the Mind: Neuroevolutionary Origins of Human Emotions [New York: W.W. Norton, 2012]). Both Damasio and neuroscientist Joseph LeDoux differentiate emotion from feeling (i.e., consciousness of emotion) together with the realization that the luxury of feeling cannot be afforded if the circumstances are too stressful (inhibition), laying the conceptual groundwork for a neuroscience of defence (Damasio, The Feeling of What Happens; Joseph LeDoux, Anxious: Using the Brain to Understand and Treat Fear and Anxiety [New York: Penguin Random House, 2015]).

8. Michael Resnick, Marjorie Ireland, and Iris Borowsky, "Youth violence perpetration: What protects? What predicts? Findings from the National Longitudinal Study of Adolescent Health," Journal of Adolescent Health: Official Publication of the Society for Adolescent Medicine 35 (2004): 424.

9. Emma Werner and Ruth S. Smith, Overcoming the Odds: High Risk Children from Birth to Adulthood (New York: Cornell University Press, 1992).

10. In a National Longitudinal Study on Adolescent Health, Michael Resnick and his colleagues found that the single most significant protective factor against emotional distress in a sample of over 90,000 adolescents in the United States was a strong caring relationship with an adult (Resnick, Ireland, and Borowsky, "Youth violence perpetration").

In Emma Werner and Ruth Smith's 30-year longitudinal research study on resilient children on the Hawaiian island of Kauai, one-third of the children who faced poverty, mental health, or addictions in their families were emotionally healthy and socially successful despite their impoverished upbringing; the significant difference with this group was that they had strong caring attachments with emotionally healthy substitute adults, including grandparents, or in schools and church communities (Werner and Smith, Overcoming the Odds). The research on resilience overwhelmingly points to strong adult relationships as having a protective factor in emotional and social well-being.

Chapter 7: Tears and Tantrums: Understanding Frustration and Aggression

1. Charles Dickens, Great Expectations (1861; New York: Rinehart, 1949).

2. Rosemarie Sokol Chang and Nicholas S. Thompson, "Whines, cries, and motherese: Their relative power to distract," *Journal of Social, Evolutionary, and Cultural Psychology* 5 (2011): 131–41.

3. Gordon Neufeld, *Making Sense of Preschoolers*, course (Neufeld Institute, Vancouver, BC, 2013), http://neufeldinstitute.org/course/making-sense-of-preschoolers/.

4. Aletha Solter, "Understanding tears and tantrums," *Young Children* 47, no. 4 (1992): 64–68.

5. William H. Frey and Muriel Langseth, *Crying: The Mystery of Tears* (Minneapolis, MN: Winston Press, 1985).

6. Ad Vingerhoets, *Why Only Humans Weep: Unravelling the Mysteries of Tears* (Oxford: Oxford University Press, 2013).

7. Rosalind Wiseman, *Masterminds and Wingmen: Helping Your Son Cope with Schoolyard Power, Locker-Room Tests, Girlfriends, and the New Rules of Boy World* (New York: Harmony Books, 2013).

8. Vingerhoets, *Why Only Humans Weep*.

9. William Blake, "Auguries of Innocence" (c. 1803).

10. Oren Hasson, "Emotional tears as biological signals," *Evolutionary Psychology* 7 (2009): 363–70.

Chapter 8: Alarmed by Disconnection: Bedtime, Separation, and Anxiety

1. Maurice Sendak, *Where the Wild Things Are* (New York: HarperCollins, 1963), p. 30.

2. Joseph E. LeDoux, *The Emotional Brain: The Mysterious Underpinnings of Emotional Life* (New York: Simon & Schuster, 1996).

3. John Bowlby, *Separation: Anxiety and Anger* (New York: Basic Books, 1973); Rollo May, *The Meaning of Anxiety* (New York: Ronald Press, 1950).

4. Thomas Lewis, Fari Amini, and Richard Lannon, *A General Theory of Love* (New York: Random House, 2000).

5. Bowlby, *Separation*.

6. S. Pathak and B.D. Perry, "Anxiety disorders," in C. Edward Coffey and Roger A. Brumback, eds., *Pediatric Neuropsychiatry* (Philadelphia: Lippincott Williams & Wilkins, 2006); Joseph E. LeDoux, *Anxious: Using the Brain to Understand and Treat Fear and Anxiety* (New York: Viking, 2015).

7. Pathak and Perry, "Anxiety disorders."

8. Timothy J. Owens and Sandra L. Hofferth, *Children at the Millennium: Where Have We Come from, Where Are We Going?* (Amsterdam: JAI, 2001).

Chapter 9: "You're Not the Boss of Me": Understanding Resistance and Opposition

1. Virginia Woolf, "The leaning tower," in *Collected Essays* (New York: Harcourt, Brace & World, 1967).

2. E.J. Lieberman, *Acts of Will: The Life and Work of Otto Rank* (Amherst: University of Massachusetts Press, 1993); E.J. Lieberman, "Rankian will," *American Journal of Psychoanalysis* 72 (2012): 320–25.

Along with Jung and Adler, Otto Rank was considered one of Freud's closest and brightest followers. Rank grew to disagree with Freud on the importance of the Oedipal complex, and many of his views were considered deviant. Rank saw the separation between mother, father, and child at birth as a critical focus in the development of self, guilt, and anxiety.

Rank was also concerned with an absence of will in Freudian therapy. He argued that individuals were capable of conscious will that brought with it guilt and anxiety. The capacity to say "no," or counterwill, was key in child development and was often diminished by adults, if not cultures. Ira Progroff wrote, "The life will as conceived by Rank is the vital force with which that potentiality is expressed and fulfilled in the world" (*The Death and Rebirth of Psychology: An Integrative Evaluation of Freud, Adler, Jung, and Rank and the Impact of Their Insights on Modern Man* [New York: McGraw-Hill, 1956], p. 207). The idea of a conscious will and resistance as a positive force underlying individuation and autonomy was not supported by Rank's psychoanalytic counterparts, and he was ostracized. In 1926 he dissociated himself from the psychoanalytic society, and his honorary membership was revoked in 1930.

See also Claude Barbre, "Confusion of wills: Otto Rank's contribution to an understanding of childism," *American Journal of Psychoanalysis* 72 (2012): 409–17; Fay B. Kargf, *The Psychology and Psychotherapy of Otto Rank: An Historical and Comparative Introduction* (New York: Philosophical Library, 1953); Esther Menaker, *Otto Rank: A Rediscovered Legacy* (New York: Columbia University Press, 1982).

3. Lieberman, "Rankian will."

4. Albert Pepitone, Clark McCauley, and Peirce Hammond, "Change in attractiveness of forbidden toys as a function of severity of threat," *Journal of Experimental*

Social Psychology 3 (1967): 221–29.

5. Mark R. Lepper, "Undermining children's intrinsic interest with extrinsic reward: A test of the 'overjustification' hypothesis," *Journal of Personality and Social Psychology* 28 (1973): 129–37.

6. Alfie Kohn, *Punished by Rewards: The Trouble with Gold Stars, Incentive Plans, A's, Praise, and Other Bribes* (Boston: Houghton Mifflin, 1993).

7. D.W. Winnicott, Clare Winnicott, Ray Shepherd, and Madeleine Davis, *Home Is Where We Start From: Essays by a Psychoanalyst* (New York: W.W. Norton, 1986).

Chapter 10: Discipline for the Immature: Buying Time for the Child to Grow Up

1. D.W. Winnicott, *Talking to Parents* (Reading, MA: Addison-Wesley, 1993), p. 86.

2. Gordon Neufeld, *Making Sense of Discipline*, course (Neufeld Institute, Vancouver, BC, 2011), http://neufeldinstitute.org/course/making-sense-of-discipline/; Daniel J. Siegel and Tina Payne Bryson, *No-Drama Discipline: The Whole-Brain Way to Calm the Chaos and Nurture Your Child's Developing Mind* (New York: Bantam Books, 2014).

3. Sara H. Konrath, Edward H. O'Brien, and Courtney Hsing, "Changes in dispositional empathy in American college students over time: A meta-analysis," *Personality and Social Psychology Review* 15 (2011): 180–98.

Chapter 11: How Young Children Grow Adults Up

1. "Dis-moi qui tu aimes, je te dirai qui tu es": Arsène Houssaye, *Le roi Voltaire* (Paris: Michel Lévy, 1858), p. 182.

Index

Figures that are images are indicated by page numbers in italics.
Endnotes are indicated by page numbers followed by "n" and a note number.

adaptive process, 20–22, *21*, 166–70
ADHD (attention-deficit/hyperactivity disorder), 42, 271n29
agendas, 215
aggression, 156, 170–74. *See also* frustration
agitation, *see* anxiety
alarm, feelings of, 138
alarm-based discipline, 228–30
alarming experiences, 115
alarm problems, 108. *See also* anxiety
alarm systems, 179–80, 225–26, 228–29, 231
Alliance for Childhood, 66
alpha instincts, in adults, 46, 104, 105–6
alpha problems, in children: introduction to, 101–3, 107–8; and alarming experiences, 115; and anxiety, 108, 185; and bullying, 114; characteristics of, 108; contributing factors to, 110, 116; and counterwill, 206; difficulty in determining, 109; and egalitarian parenting, 112–13; and

fostering child's dependence on parent, 117–18, 121–22; and frustrations, 151, 165; and hierarchical relationships, 119–20; and parents' background, 111; parents' strong alpha presence for, 116–17; and passive parenting, 112; and play, 63; proactive meeting of needs for, 118–19; problems resulting from, 108–9; and providing opportunities for alpha expression, 119; reactions to, 121; and sensitive children, 114–15; and separation anxiety, 113–14; strategies for, 115–16, 122; and taking charge of decisions and circumstances, 120–21
anxiety, 184–85. *See also* separation
attachment: introduction to, 75–76; alpha instincts in, 104, 105–6; and brain function, 77; bridging for, 189–90; as context for rest, 8; and counterwill, 204–5, 216; for creating mature social beings, 23–24; definition of, 77; dependent instincts in, 104–5; development from, 94; and following orders, 105; ideas for contact and closeness, 95; importance of for children, 16–17, 77–78,